www.b a ord ok/

D1761207

Health Informatics

Stephen Goundrey-Smith

Principles of Electronic Prescribing

Second Edition

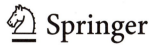 Springer

Stephen Goundrey-Smith, MSc
Cert Clin Pharm, MRPharmS
SGS PharmaSolutions, Chedworth
Gloucestershire
UK

ISBN 978-1-4471-4044-3 2nd edition   ISBN 978-1-4471-4045-0 2nd edition   (eBook)
ISBN 978-1-84800-234-0 1st edition   ISBN 978-1-84800-235-7 1st edition   (eBook)
DOI 10.1007/978-1-4471-4045-0
Springer Dordrecht Heidelberg New York London

Library of Congress Control Number: 2012939967

First published in 2008

Printed on acid-free paper

Springer is part of Springer Science+Business Media (www.springer.com)

Preface

This book is the result of several years of reflection and work in the area of electronic prescribing and medicines management. It represents a major project for me, as a pharmacist, a health informatician and as a writer. However, in my experience, major undertakings such as this are rarely the sole work of one person. I would therefore like to make a number of acknowledgements, and to thank a number of people whose assistance and support has been invaluable in the production of this book.

I would like to thank those hospital staff who were willing to be interviewed and to share their experiences of electronic medicines management with me:

- Pete MacGuinness, Senior Clinical Pharmacist at the Shrewsbury and Telford NHS Trust.
- Daphne Hitchman at the Royal Hampshire County Hospital, at Winchester.

I am also grateful to those who were of assistance with certain sections of the book.

- Hillary Judd and colleagues from First Databank Europe Ltd, for their input in the area of data support for electronic prescribing.
- Joan Povey from JAC Computer Services Ltd for providing screen views of the JAC electronic prescribing medicines administration module.

I am especially indebted, however, to those people with whom I have worked most closely on the electronic prescribing and pharmacy IT agendas over the past ten years. In a sense, my expertise reflects theirs. They are (in no particular order):

- Former colleagues and associates from iSOFT – George Brown, Tom Bolitho, Clive Spindley, Tim Botten, Sue Braithwaite, Julie Randall and Raghu Kumar
- Heidi Wright from the Royal Pharmaceutical Society and Lindsay McClure from the Pharmaceutical Services Negotiating Committee.
- Fellow members for the Guild of Healthcare Pharmacists/United Kingdom Clinical Pharmacy Association (UKCPA) IT Interest Group Committee

I would also like to thank:

- Eric Smith for his work on illustrations
- Eddie Smith for his comments concerning pathology systems
- Grant Weston and colleagues at Springer for their editorial support.

Above all, I am grateful to my family – Sally, Edward, Archie, Sam and Emily – for their support.

Contents

Chapter 1
Philosophical and Social Framework of Electronic Medicines Management

Introduction

Electronic prescribing involves the use of computer systems to facilitate the prescription, supply and administration of medicines within a hospital. Electronic prescribing (EP) systems are able to capture a full prescribing history for a patient in a transferable manner, and open up the potential for use of databases and decision support tools to assist the prescriber in medicine selection.

Over the last 10–20 years, EP systems have been developed and used in a number of countries around the world, but their use is by no means widespread. Currently, in the United Kingdom, only a handful of acute hospitals have full electronic prescribing systems throughout the hospital. There are, however, further hospitals with electronic prescribing in certain wards and specialties only. Electronic prescribing systems – and in particular, computerized decision support tools to aid prescribing – have been pioneered in the United States, and there is much research documentation on their use in a US context. Nevertheless EP systems have still not been widely adopted in the US, for various reasons. In addition, electronic prescribing and clinical decision support tools are increasingly being implemented in Australia and in European countries other than the UK (Fig. 1.1).

However, due to sociopolitical developments on a global scale, healthcare providers around the world are increasingly concerned with cost-effectiveness, the increased likelihood of litigation and the need for clinical governance, quality and transparency in healthcare processes. Consequently, there will be an increasing emphasis on the clinical application of information technology to help healthcare providers streamline their business processes to achieve outcome targets and to optimize care quality and cost-effectiveness. An area of healthcare where there is a critical need to use IT for these purposes is the prescribing and supply of medicines in secondary care.

Use of departmental systems to manage the discrete activities of particular departments or specialisms in hospitals is now well-established. For many years, hospitals around the world have been using systems to process patient data, manage

S. Goundrey-Smith, *Principles of Electronic Prescribing*, Health Informatics, DOI 10.1007/978-1-4471-4045-0_1, © Springer-Verlag London 2012

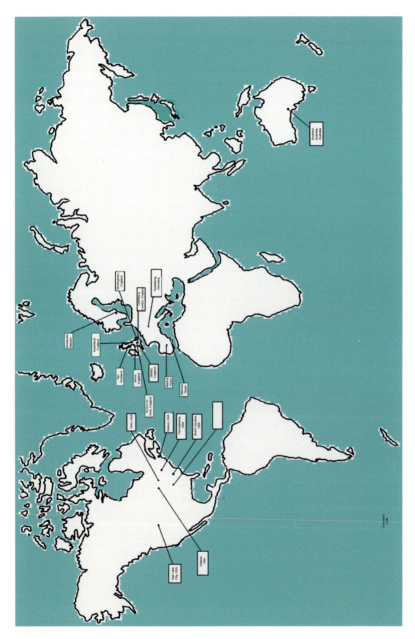

Fig. 1.1 Worldwide experience of hospital electronic prescribing. Centers with published experience of EP system implementation in secondary care (For full details, see Appendix 1)

clinics or treatment episodes, and to create and communicate orders (e.g. radiology or pathology orders). These would include <u>patient administration systems (PAS)</u> to manage admissions and <u>discharge</u> and to facilitate the <u>patient pathway</u>, or "patient journey" in <u>secondary care</u>, and systems for pathology laboratory and pharmacy management. However, the area of electronic prescribing and clinical medicines management is one where the adoption of technology is at an earlier stage.

There are now compelling – but, at points, contestable – data concerning the role of EP systems in <u>risk reduction</u> and optimizing <u>business processes</u> in hospitals. There are also clear benefits for the use of well-structured and maintained clinical decision support systems for the prescribing process. The benefits data for both EP systems and clinical decision support tools will be discussed in subsequent chapters. For these reasons, there is an increasing interest in the benefits of EP systems from both healthcare professionals and healthcare provider managers, and there is likely to be continued growth in adoption of EP systems over the next 10 years.

Elsewhere in <u>Europe</u>, <u>regional and national healthcare IT programmes</u> have been established to address population healthcare issues.[1] In the US, systems have been established by the major healthcare insurance providers to optimize the quality and cost-effectiveness of treatment, especially for long term conditions [3]. The <u>Connecting for Health</u> (CfH) national IT programme for the <u>National Health Service (NHS)</u> in <u>England,</u> which ran from 2002 to 2011 did not deliver a national EP solution for hospitals in England, as originally envisaged. However, the CfH E-prescribing programme has provided methodology advice and research resources for hospital EP implementers [4], and has had a valuable coordinating role helping hospitals in England share implementation experience with some of the EP systems that are already commercially available.[2]

In any given health economy, a broad constituency of professionals are involved in the design, implementation, management and maintenance of electronic prescribing systems, depending on the technology employed, the structure and organisation of the healthcare system concerned, and the roles of the different professionals within the system. This would include <u>healthcare professionals</u> (doctors, nurses, pharmacists and other healthcare professions), healthcare managers and administrators, IT specialists from within the health system or <u>software vendors</u>, drug data suppliers and other <u>stakeholders</u>, such as government <u>regulatory bodies</u> or the <u>pharmaceutical industry</u>.

This book will discuss issues associated with <u>secondary care</u> electronic prescribing systems and clinical decision support to date, the basic principles of design and implementation of these systems, and how their design and configuration can impact on <u>benefits realisation</u>, <u>hospital workflow</u> and <u>clinical practice</u>. While the book

---

[1] For example, the Umbrian regional healthcare system in Italy (see Barbarito [1]) and the Stockholm Regional Drug Prescribing System in Sweden (See Sjoborg et al. [2]).

[2] The NHS Connecting for Health e-prescribing programme has had an important role in sharing the experience of previous implementations – see http://www.connectingforhealth.nhs.uk/systemsandservices/eprescribing/challenges.

explores the current benefits and potential role of EP systems in hospitals, and describes <u>interfaces</u> with other <u>secondary care</u> systems (for example <u>pharmacy systems</u> and <u>pathology systems</u>), discussion of primary care IT systems for medicines management – in particular, the <u>electronic transfer of prescriptions (eTP)</u> in community pharmacy – is outwith the scope of the book. There is, however, an expectation that, in future, <u>secondary care</u> and <u>primary care</u> systems will be able to communicate with each other.

This book will necessarily refer to the published literature to illustrate the recognized benefits of EP systems and the potential applications of such systems, described in each chapter. Since the first edition of the book, a greater body of research literature has become available, with work on clinical decision support methodology, paediatric EP processes, user perceptions of EP systems, together with new material on risk management and error reduction. This second edition incorporates the findings of this research but, as with the first edition, does not attempt to provide an exhaustive review or quantitative analysis of published studies.

This chapter will set the scene by exploring some of the social, political and philosophical issues that attend the use of electronic systems in healthcare, and in particular, electronic prescribing systems.

Definitions and Terminology

Since electronic systems for medicine prescribing have been developed independently in different countries, under the auspices of different healthcare systems, it is inevitable that there will be variations in terminology. Furthermore, terms that are not synonymous may be used interchangeably or in an indiscriminate manner.

A recent UK <u>definition of</u> *electronic prescribing* is as follows:

> The utilisation of electronic systems to facilitate and enhance the communication of a prescription or medicine order, aiding the choice, administration and supply of a medicine through knowledge and <u>decision support</u>, and providing a robust audit trail for the entire medicines use process
> NHS Connecting for Health [5]

This is a useful working definition for an EP system because it takes into account the capacity of an EP system to add value to the patient's <u>prescribing history</u> through use of clinical <u>decision support</u> tools, and also the process of storage and communication of medicine orders. It is an appropriate description of some of the EP systems in current use in the UK. It is also a suitable definition for many of the US EP systems that are available at present.

However, in the US, the term *Computerized Physician Order Entry (CPOE)* is often used in the literature to describe computer applications that are used for electronic prescribing. This term is often used synonymously with *electronic prescribing*. However, *CPOE* is a broader term which can encompass the transmission of other clinical order types, such as <u>pathology tests</u> or <u>radiology tests</u>, as well as medication orders. However, when applied to medication orders, *CPOE* only addresses the prescribing element of the medication use process [6], together with the electronic transmission of the medicine order. Strictly speaking, the term *CPOE* does not embrace the <u>database</u> and decision support elements of an EP system, which are regarded by many commentators as an essential aspect of an EP system.

In the US, the provision of medication in response to prescriber orders and the management of the supply of medicines is the role of *pharmacy information systems* [7]. These systems are designed to manage information relating to the use of medicines in patient care and include functionality for online order entry, pharmacist review, medication profiles, label printing, stock/inventory control and reporting (medication use reports, dispensing reports etc.). Since some *pharmacy information systems* may be used to facilitate electronic prescribing, with online order entry and, in some cases, clinical decision support tools, some commentators consider them as electronic prescribing applications. However, this is in contrast to the UK, where there is a more clear demarcation between <u>pharmacy systems</u>, which are well-developed and universally used, and electronic prescribing systems, which are still in their infancy.

In Europe, the <u>European Committee for Standardisation</u> has defined electronic prescriptions in terms of the exchange of prescription messages between <u>prescribers</u> and <u>dispensers</u>, and between healthcare providers and official authorities as permitted by national regulations.[3]

This definition focuses on the dissemination of prescription information between stakeholder organisations, following recognized messaging conventions and in accordance with national laws, thus reflecting the EU emphasis on removing <u>barriers to commerce</u> across the <u>European Union</u>. It does not mention clinical decision support, and is concerned with the business and commercial aspects, rather than the clinical aspects, of the medicines use process.

The definitions and terms used have different emphases and, when used correctly, reflect different aspects of the whole medicines use process. Overall, it is clear from a discussion of the terminology that EP is a complex discipline, the success of which relies on the successful interplay of system design, data support and clinical practice.

In addition, the term *electronic medicines management* should be considered. *Electronic medicines management* is a broader term than *electronic prescribing* since it encompasses all medicine related activities – including selection, <u>supply</u>, <u>medicines administration</u> and <u>monitoring</u> of medicine use – not just the act of prescribing. It is therefore a useful description of many contemporary EP systems, which are comprehensive in their scope, and are designed to support and manage all medicines-related activities in a hospital. However, the term *medicines management* is one that has largely been coined by the UK pharmacy profession and has little currency outside the UK and outside the pharmacy profession.

---

[3] European Committee for Standardisation. European PreStandard (ENV) 13607. Health Informatics. Messages for the exchange of information on medicine prescriptions.

As well as definitions of the overall process of electronic prescribing, it is recognized that the descriptors and nomenclatures used within the EP systems must conform to recognized standards in order for the systems to be internally consistent in their operation and intraoperable with other systems. Controlled terminologies, as they relate to EP systems in particular, will be discussed in the chapter on data support. However, it has to be recognized that the major harmonisation endeavours for healthcare IT – for example, Health Level Seven (HL7) and the International Standards Organisation (ISO) TC 215 – seek to address process issues beyond the prescribing of medicines in a clinical scenario. So, for example, the ISO TC 215 standard for Identification of medicinal products (structures and controlled vocabularies for ingredients (substances))[4] lists international pharmacovigilance (reporting of side effects of drugs), clinical trials, product regulatory approval and environmental protection/toxicology as business use cases for controlled vocabulary for medicines, as well as electronic prescribing.

The Benefits of Automated Systems

In the earliest days of computer technology, automated systems were developed in order to store and retrieve information. With the advent of solid state technology, where for the first time it was possible to build computers that were powerful enough to handle large volumes of data with optimal speed, but small enough to be of practical use in a working environment, organisations began to see the potential of computer-based systems to replace bulky paper records.

Computer-based systems also bring the possibility of fast and accurate retrieval of information, based on appropriate indexing and coding methodology. There is also the potential to post messages against certain records according to keywords and other attributes, which is potentially useful in clinical applications. Indexing and coding can present procedural issues in the design of a simple database, concerning classification, accessioning etc.; in the area of medicines and therapeutics information, the use of indexing methodology to provide clinical decision support is potentially a very complex – and critical – science. Data structures and coding systems for medicines data will be discussed in detail in a later chapter, together with use cases and known problem scenarios.

A review of experience of EP applications in the UK [8] has indicated that electronic prescribing implementations have resulted in the following benefits:

- Availability of a fully electronic prescribing history.
- Improvement in legibility and completeness of prescriptions.
- Improvement of hospital business processes due to electronic dissemination of prescriptions.

---

[4] International Standards Organisation. Health Informatics – Identification of medicinal products – Structures and controlled vocabularies for Ingredients (Substances) ISO TC 215/WG 6 N 549.

- Availability of electronic <u>decision support</u> tools at the point of prescribing.
- Comprehensive <u>audit trail</u> of prescribing decisions made.
- Reduction in the rate of <u>medication errors</u>.

Some of these benefits have also been reflected in the major quantitative studies of EP systems in the United States. These benefits will be discussed in detail in subsequent chapters.

The benefits of EP systems are far-reaching in significance, in terms of effects on <u>risk management</u> and <u>risk reduction</u>, and also <u>financial cost</u>. However, it is acknowledged by experts in the field that realisation of these benefits is dependent on <u>system design</u> [9]. Given the likely growth of interest in <u>electronic medicines management</u>, a discussion of design issues with electronic medicines management systems, and their impact on benefits, will be timely for the many groups of professionals likely to be involved.

Automated systems offer advantages over traditional paper-based systems in three main areas:

- <u>Accuracy</u> – automated systems can support the consistent use of medicine nomenclature, the accurate recording, display and transmission of prescription information, and the accurate display of clinical warnings as a result of a logical system of trigger points. In short, EP systems automate <u>repetitive processes</u> or <u>monotonous processes</u> which are prone to <u>human error</u> when carried out manually [10]. Thus automated systems are able to contribute to <u>risk management</u> objectives in hospital prescribing.
- <u>Standardisation of data</u> – automated systems allow patient data to be captured and stored according to standard formats and conventions. This facilitates the electronic transfer of patient data, and the production of comprehensive <u>management reports</u>. The production of <u>management reports</u> by hospitals and healthcare providers is an issue of great political significance in many healthcare economies where there is a need for governments and the public to be aware of healthcare issues and outcomes. However, reporting is an area of clinical IT where there are often many methodological and technical obstacles to be surmounted. It is hoped that EP systems in development will address important deliverables in management reporting. However, in standardizing patient data, electronic systems therefore have the capacity for what has been described as <u>"mass customisation"</u> [10]. In healthcare terms, this means that, although the system handles large amounts of patient data, it is able to produce an individual care plan based on the specific personal requirements of each patient.
- Facilitating <u>changes in working practices</u> – automated systems have the capacity to process prescription information accurately and at scale, and are able to facilitate the display of that information in different contexts, according to <u>system design</u> and hardware availability. They are therefore able to make possible new ways of working for individuals and organisations. Because the system takes care of the routine recording, computational and transmission aspects of prescription information management, organisation processes may be restructured so that health professionals can engage with <u>near-patient clinical activities</u>, which

Fig. 1.2 The relationship between the EP system, the healthcare provider organization and the state

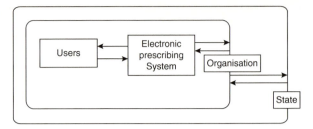

require intuitive human qualities. Nevertheless, while re-engineering of business processes may be possible with automated systems, it may not always be desirable, and the objective of software design may be simply to automate and improve the efficiency of existing working processes (Fig. 1.2).

Electronic Prescribing and the Individual

Given that electronic systems have the potential to improve <u>health outcomes</u> and <u>care quality</u>, through increased accuracy of prescription information management and dissemination, and to revolutionize working practices, the implementation of an EP system may have a significant impact on individual users – the healthcare professionals involved with the prescription, supply and administration of medicines. The introduction of an EP system will also have consequences for the working lives of hospital managers, healthcare informaticians and IT professionals and other health provider staff who are not patient-facing.

Many individual healthcare professionals will appreciate the potential benefits of an EP system; they will see the potential for a system to improve health outcomes and reduce risk in their particular area of practice. This will be especially the case for consultant medical staff whose performance may well be monitored using the <u>health outcome</u> and <u>care quality</u> information for their patient list. However, in an increasingly regulated healthcare environment, other healthcare professionals will see the value of EP systems in helping them to achieve performance objectives and to comply with ethical, legal and professional requirements [11]. Some healthcare professionals, however, may be concerned about adverse effects on their sphere of practice, with the political and <u>litigation</u> implications that those adverse effects might entail. For this reason, they may be concerned about the capacity for electronic systems to generate new and uncharacterized errors, which is well-recognized in the literature [12].

Furthermore, an individual's attitude towards the implementation of an electronic system is often not related to whether or not they are familiar with the documented research evidence for the use of such systems. This suggests that factors other than system knowledge and familiarity affect a person's attitude to the introduction on an electronic system.

An <u>automated system</u> may introduce a new way of doing one or more <u>business processes</u> within an organisation, and therefore bring about <u>changes in working</u>

practices. There is therefore a requirement that individuals are trained on the new system and, as mentioned earlier, a new system can facilitate new ways of working in more general terms.

A number of factors influence an individual's willingness to engage with a new way of working, and their resistance to change. These include:

- An individual's personal response to innovations and changes of any kind. In marketing theory, it is recognized that, by character, some individuals are innovators, some early adopters, some early majority, some late majority and some laggards [13]. For an information product, it is known that the proportions of these groups are 2.5%, 13.5%, 34%, 34% and 16% respectively.
- An individual's personal view of technology. Some people may be "technophobes" for any number of reasons, such as a bad experience with a previous computer system, either at work or at home, or a feeling of disempowerment because, in the consumer world, large corporate bodies are using IT systems aggressively to manipulate their customer base and achieve their commercial goals.
- The threat of a change to an individual's status or position within the organisation. With an EP system, some people in the organisation – in particular, lower paid staff such as pharmacy support staff and healthcare assistants – may feel that their jobs are at risk, because of automation. EP and pharmacy automation generally do not lead to reduction in posts, however, as will be discussed in Chap. 3. In addition, some people may feel that the change in working practice is one way of another professional group exercising power over them, or that they are having to do extra work so that another professional group can reap the benefits.
- An individual's bewilderment and confusion concerning the exact role and operation of a new system. It is to be hoped that this barrier to successful implementation can be at least partly removed by a thorough programme of training and orientation. Many reports of EP implementations stress the importance of appropriate training for system users.

As well as the implementation process itself, the routine use of an EP system may have a profound influence on the working processes of individual healthcare professionals. Conversely, the success of the system may be influenced by the way in which individual health professionals work with it. A number of factors can be identified.

- A functionally-rich EP system will make a larger amount of clinical data available to healthcare professionals at the point of patient care [14]. This may necessitate the acquisition of new skills in clinical data evaluation, which may have implications for continuing professional development. This may also lead to a state of "information saturation" for busy health professionals, which could cause increased levels of stress in daily practice.
- An EP system may well enable new and unfamiliar ways of working. These may be beneficial to health professions in the long run, but may be stressful in the short term. Moreover, without good management, especially proactive change

management, with the introduction of clear procedures, new ways of working may initially introduce more critical incidents that they resolve.

- An EP system may be used to facilitate new ways of doing critical incident based continuing professional development (CPD). This is beneficial at a time when health professionals are increasingly regulated in terms of the amount and format of CPD and the use of CPD as the basis for professional accreditation. This area will be explored in greater depth in Chap. 6.
- It is recognized that people are less likely to question the accuracy and authenticity of information when it is displayed on a computer system, than when it is recorded in medical notes or on a drug chart, perhaps in a poorly legible or ambiguous manner. This effect may lead to complacency in clinical practice in future, when EP systems are universally available, where the assumption that "the computer is always right" leads to errors and near misses. Clinical users will need to gain confidence in the due diligence process surrounding the implementation of EP software, but at the same time will need to retain a level of vigilance when presented with data by an EP system. An EP system will never replace the clinical judgement of an experienced health professional.
- As mentioned previously, decision support functions within an EP system are an important way in which the EP system "adds value" to the prescribing process. However, as experience with currently-used GP, hospital pharmacy and community pharmacy systems suggests, systems often provide a highly detailed level of decision support on a range of parameters – sensitivity checking, drug interactions, drug disease interactions, contraindications etc. – but they may not be configured to display warnings according to clinical significance, or to display only the warnings that are relevant to the patient in question. In some cases, with drug interaction warnings, a system might display all reciprocal warnings; for example, the system will display two warning messages, showing that there is a drug interaction between aspirin and warfarin, and also between warfarin and aspirin The result is that, on prescribing a medicine, an EP system user may be presented with an exhaustive list of warnings, many of which are duplicated, or are of questionable relevance, and will be required to click an acknowledgement of each one. This can lead to what has been termed as "warning fatigue", where the user becomes inattentive concerning the warnings displayed, due to the presence of irrelevant warnings, and will inadvertently ignore a significant warning. Warning fatigue is an important cause of decision support failure in EP systems; data providers, system implementers and researchers are undertaking ongoing research into the nature of the problem, and its possible solutions by making changes to the data structure or the user interface. The problems associated with decision support in EP systems will be discussed fully in Chap. 5.

The introduction of an EP system may have consequences for hospital managers and health provider staff who are not patient-facing and who would not be routine users of an EP system. Many healthcare managers will understandably see the successful implementation and use of an EP system as:

(a) an important factor in the reduction of clinical and organisational risks, and thus the risk of <u>litigation</u>;
(b) a means of improving <u>clinical governance</u> and <u>information governance</u> so that hospital management has accurate information on actual <u>health outcomes</u> in the organization, which is held as securely as possible.

Nevertheless, some managers will see an EP system as a "quick fix" for one or more longstanding problems in the organisation. These managers are likely to become frustrated when they realize that the process of change itself is often a slow one, and will become impatient at the amount of low-level detail that needs to be considered with an EP system implementation. Other <u>hospital managers</u> may see the implementation of an EP system as a means of achieving their targets at the expense of the working practices of other professional groups in the hospital, or may see the system as a way of imposing an organisational or ideological agenda on other groups of staff, which will bring them into conflict with one or more other groups of staff.

Electronic Prescribing and the Organisation

As is clear from the previous section, the issues and problems that affect an individual when an EP system is implemented are inextricably linked with the issues that face the organisation as a whole, when a system is introduced. An organisation is, to a greater or lesser extent, the sum of its individuals. This section examines some of the organisational issues facing hospitals and other secondary care health providers when an EP system is implemented.

The earliest prescribing and medical information systems in the UK were designed for use in general practice and their use in <u>primary care</u> has become widespread, following the introduction of <u>Read codes</u>, which enabled the common classification of medical terms for audit purposes [15], which in turn facilitated the electronic storage and transmission of patient information, including information about their prescriptions. <u>General practice (GP) systems</u> have been on the market for over 30 years and have adapted to changes in medical practice in primary care during that time. Furthermore, the databases provided by leading <u>third-party data suppliers</u> were originally designed to meet the needs of primary care computer systems; primary care systems suppliers are still the chief consumers of <u>third party drug databases.</u>

This begs the important question: why has electronic prescribing and medicine/prescribing information management not developed in a similar way in secondary care? Why is EP largely still in its infancy in secondary care health providers around the world, when the technologies to enable it have existed for some time?

The lack of adoption of EP systems in secondary care is, in many respects, due to organisational issues. A primary care medical practice – even a large one, such as a ten-partner practice in a large town – represents a discrete working unit, where practice personnel are expected to work as a team, and the partners and practice manager have control over the systems in place within the practice. In this environment, the choice, implementation and maintenance of an electronic system is a relatively easy matter. <u>Stakeholder engagement</u> ("buy-in") with the new system is easier to achieve with a small, well-defined practice team, the installation of the system can be project managed in a relatively controlled manner, and the logistics of training personnel does not present major problems.

It is a different scenario with an average acute hospital. Hospitals are larger, comprising of a number of distinct wards and departments. There are a range of clinical and non-clinical professions working in a hospital and, historically, the working practices of each profession have been governed by the profession itself, rather than engagement in multidisciplinary teams, and this fosters professional segregation and rivalry, rather than multidisciplinary working. In many hospitals, the hospital management structures are heterogenous, at best, and may be unable to hold together the divergent professional interests and departmental agendas in the organisation.

From a political perspective, this diffuse organisational structure considerably increases the problems associated the change management required to introduce a new system across the hospital. When there are a number of distinct and separate stakeholders, it is essential for implementers to secure <u>stakeholder engagement</u>, and ensure that all professional agendas are acknowledged. Failure to do this can lead to an important stakeholder being disenfranchised, with disastrous consequences for the implementation project. Moreover, the implementation of a new system may exacerbate existing rivalries between professional groups. This is especially the case if one professional group has a greater role in the implementation than another.

The implementation and roll-out of an EP system within a hospital represents a major business project, and will require formal project management and project structure – the standard methodology for which is PRINCE 2, in the UK healthcare environment. A clinical IT project will require engagement with stakeholders, process redesign and training of users in the new system. This in itself will be stressful for those directly involved in the project team. Secondly, it is recognized that the most successful EP implementations in hospitals are ones where every effort has been made to engage all stakeholders – doctors, pharmacists, nurses, managers, IT staff and others – and to encourage them to take ownership of the new system [16]. Conversely, it is often the case that, if one particular professional group drives the project, according to its own agenda, the implementation is less likely to be successful.

Because of the segregation of the professions in the NHS, historically healthcare applications used in the NHS have been designed for use in a particular department, to manage a discrete, well-defined process. This approach was taken with both <u>pharmacy systems</u> and <u>pathology systems</u>, which were the earliest systems to be implemented in NHS hospitals. Moreover, such systems often began as "home grown", designed by innovative health professionals, with IT expertise.[5]

---

[5] This approach has been taken in electronic medicines management with the eSCRIPT transcription system used by the Shrewsbury and Telford Hospitals NHS Trust in the UK.

Consequently, IT systems in the NHS have in the past been subject to "silo" development in individual departments – i.e. as separate systems with no ability for interaction or integration with other departmental systems. As time has gone by, concerns have been raised about the ability of these systems to share patient data throughout the hospital, the capacity of the different systems to introduce inconsistencies in data handling, and the difficulties of configuring these departmental systems to operate in other hospitals.

Software vendors have responded in two main ways to the issue of "silo" development. Some have provided appropriate interfaces so that their system is intraoperable with other hospital systems. Thus, the vendor of an EP system would typically need to provide interfaces with the hospital's patient administration system (PAS), to gain access to patient demographic data, and with the hospital's pharmacy system, to allow seamless transfer of prescription information to the pharmacy department. However, such interfaces are problematic in that they are often complex to build and require thorough testing. Other software suppliers have developed an enterprise wide system with different modules to manage different hospital processes, which can be implemented at different times. For example, the Winchester TMS system, and the Meditech system used in the Wirral and Burton on Trent hospitals worked on this basis.

Furthermore, one of the objectives of large regional or national IT programmes is often to surmount issues relating to connectivity and intraoperability. This goal has been successfully achieved with regional healthcare systems implemented in Sweden, Italy and the US.

As well as the organisational issues highlighted above, there are other factors that limit implementation of EP within healthcare enterprises. These include:

- The financial cost, especially with commercial systems. This is linked with the fact that the EP software may be sold by a vendor as part of a larger integrated system, and the healthcare provider may only wish to purchase the EP component. There also
- Legal issues and due diligence process concerns of healthcare providers. These will be discussed in detail later in the chapter
- Political issues – paradoxically, one factor that limited clinical system innovation in the UK was the introduction of the Connecting for Health programme. Because of CfH, many UK NHS Trusts put a freeze on implementation of new clinical systems in the early twenty-first century, pending the introduction of CfH compliant systems. It may be argued therefore that the English national programme has stifled EP innovation [17].

In any case, the use of an EP system within a healthcare provider organization should not be considered simply as a matter of system and process, because users will react to the system in different ways. Some will find work-arounds to avoid their working practices being altered by the system, and some will "game the system" if they can – i.e. use the system in such a way that it supports their working practices. For these reasons, the operation of an EP system should take into account the human computer interface and the working practices taking place around it.

Consequently, Barber has described EP systems as a "sociotechnical system" within an organisation and has indicated that the configuration of EP systems should be considered "work in progress" throughout the life of the system, to take into account unexpected consequences arising from working practices and human interaction with the system [18].

Electronic Prescribing and the State

As mentioned earlier, electronic systems for use in healthcare applications have traditionally been developed within the UK NHS on a "silo" basis – i.e. as separate systems – where intraoperability is dependent on the resilience of hospital servers and networks, and the availability of robust interfaces with associate systems. Even with the technical ability to link systems, there may be issues with actual information exchange due to lack of standardisation of data and data structure.

The silo development of hospital systems has had profound implications for management of healthcare at government level. The duplication of basic demographic data, and the need to rekey basic patient details in certain cases, has in the past provided a huge workload burden on health providers. The use of different systems in different parts of the country means that, when an individual moves to another region, or is treated in a different hospital, their electronic patient record (EPR) has to be re-keyed on a new system, potentially introducing inconsistencies. Furthermore, if a patient is treated as an emergency away from home, their medical information stored in electronic form at their local hospital is not available to the professionals involved in the emergency situation.

In addition to issues surrounding the treatment of individual patients, silo development of systems in the health services have hindered the collation of data for public health reporting purposes. Governments need to gain an accurate picture of the health needs – and health outcomes – of the population. A well-publicized and emotive example of this in the UK, is the situation with reporting of cancer statistics, where in the past, there have been inconsistencies and gaps in information available to the Department of Health on cancer incidences and outcomes [19]. The introduction of national cancer data standards to provide a framework for reporting of cancer epidemiological data, has gone some way to resolving this issue.

There is therefore a strong political argument for the introduction of clinical IT as part of a regional or national healthcare IT programme. A larger programme has the potential to:

(a) provide seamless operation of clinical systems across the region or country and thus facilitate consistent patient care.
(b) provide standard user interfaces that are used by all health professionals; this is a factor that will reduce operational risks due to human error.
(c) provide a consistent framework for public health management reporting and clinical governance across a region or country.

As mentioned earlier in the chapter, a number of regional programmes have been implemented to a greater or lesser extent elsewhere in Europe, most notably in Sweden, and Italy. In the UK, the NHS <u>Connecting for Health</u> national IT programme ran from 2002 to 2011, with the aim of delivering a range of national healthcare IT services. While the programme delivered some useful systems, such as NHSMail and the Choose & Book primary care medical booking system, it did not fulfil its original remit of providing extensive national solutions in all areas of healthcare.

In general terms, large-scale IT projects such as this are often not successful, because they are associated with a high level of political and logistical inertia, due to the engagement of the many stakeholders involved, and the scale of the project process that has to be managed. Also, when concerns about deliverability are raised, public opinion about the programme is diminished and <u>stakeholder</u> morale is lowered, leading to a downward spiral in programme efficacy. The problem was compounded with the UK CfH project in that it was based on a three-tier system – CfH engaged a number of <u>local service providers (LSPs)</u>, who were contracted to deliver the technological infrastructure, and who had subcontracted healthcare software vendors to provide the software. This structure increased the number of stakeholders, and therefore the amount of political friction associated with the programme, and it is likely that this contributed to the inability of the programme to deliver the promised software solutions. Also, major concerns were expressed about the ability of software vendors to produce software that was fit for purpose for UK clinical use within the projected timeframe of the project.

As discussed earlier, the English national programme has slowed down EP adoption [17]. When the programme was inaugurated in 2002, a number of NHS Trusts in the UK stopped ongoing implementation projects, with the intention of adopting the CfH software when it was available. When it became clear that CfH solutions were not forthcoming, some NHS Trusts opted to implement <u>interim solutions,</u> especially in specialist areas such as oncology and radiology, which were further ahead in the CfH roadmap. These Trusts realized that there were clear managerial and clinical benefits from implementing an interim system, on the basis that they might use such a system for more than 5 years, before any national solution becomes available. Connecting for Health acknowledged this by conducting a <u>benchmarking process</u> on available <u>oncology systems</u> in 2006.

It was then recognized that electronic prescribing and medicines administration functions would not be delivered as part of a national system, and the emphasis of the CfH hospital e-prescribing programme shifted from the design and development of new, national systems, to the evaluation of EP systems that were already commercially available and providing advice on EP methodology [20].

During the latter years of the national programme, some UK healthcare providers became impatient with progress on national solutions, and chose to make their own implementations. The Royal Liverpool and Broadgreen University Hospitals Trust chose to implement a EP system independently of CfH, and therefore at its own cost, because of concern with the slowness of the national programme and in order to fit with other technical priorities in the Trust [21]. The Shrewsbury and

Telford NHS Trust implemented an <u>electronic transcribing system</u> which has been developed within the Trust, which has gone some way to meet medicines management needs in the hospital, particularly around the discharge process (Personal Communication – Pete MacGuinness, Shrewsbury & Telford NHS Trust).

The <u>United States</u> health system also faces a major challenge in the development of EP systems. An urgent priority for the US government is to manage expenditure on chronic diseases, in particular in the large proportion of low-waged Americans whose treatment is funded by the government insurance schemes <u>Medicare</u> and <u>Medicaid</u>. EP systems have the capacity to optimize cost effective medicine use but there will need to be a greater adoption of EP systems before electronic prescribing has a significant impact on prescribing in the Medicare/Medicaid populations. For this reason, recent legislation has been introduced to encourage more widespread adoption of EP systems, largely by setting standards of intraoperability across the wide range of software vendors in the US market place [3]. The current challenge in the US is the adoption of systems to manage the electronic prescribing process in the community, the automation of communications between the physician's office, the pharmacy and the pharmacy benefits management organization and, in particular, the engagement of pharmacists with this process. Two books have been published recently to outline the benefits of EP to US community-based pharmacists and to assist them with EP adoption [22, 23]. Many of the benefits appear to be similar to those seen with hospital-based electronic prescribing and, although both authors consider research conducted in hospital settings, these publications are primarily concerned with EP in the community rather than in hospitals, and will not be considered in any further detail here.

Perceptions of EP Systems

As already mentioned, the perceptions of EP systems by individual healthcare professionals and other users are key determinants of stakeholder engagement with system implementation, and the effective use of these systems, given that the EP system may be described as a "sociotechnical system". A number of studies have been conducted on staff perceptions of EP systems following their implementation, in various healthcare systems and contexts around the world.

Abdel Qader et al. [24] looked at satisfaction predictors and attitudes to EP systems among 335 doctors and 67 pharmacists in three UK hospitals. The majority of pharmacists and doctors agreed that the EP system improved the efficiency of prescribing and reduced medication errors. However, most did not believe that the EP system created more time for near patient clinical activities, or sped up the discharge process. More pharmacists than doctors believed that EP systems improved patient care, which might be because pharmacists found the use of EP systems less interruptive to their working practices than doctors did. In contrast to this study, research by Steinschaden et al. [25] and Hellstrom et al. [26] on the perceptions of EP systems of Austrian and Swedish physicians indicated that doctors believed that the systems did save time in the prescribing process. However, the differing perceptions of the time taken to prescribe using the EP system may be due to different practice contexts.

In a survey of attitudes to electronic prescribing among doctors and pharmacists in Singapore, Tan et al. [27] found that both professions generally agreed that the EP system reduced prescribing errors and interventions, and that they would not wish to return to paper-based systems. Pharmacy users in this study reported that the EP system interrupted their workflow, however.

Mehta and Onatade [28] studied the use of EP systems in detail in a telephone survey of pharmacists in seven UK hospitals (two of which were teaching hospitals). The seven hospitals used three different EP systems, all with clinical decision support functions maintained by the pharmacy department. All respondents indicated that the implementation of EP had led to changes in the pharmacy service, such as methods of medicine ordering and stock control, and also new clinically-focused roles for pharmacists. Respondents generally saw EP as a benefit, and stated that there were more advantages than disadvantages. The authors indicated that a multidisciplinary approach was needed for a successful EP implementation, together with a suitable pilot and roll-out process, and a robust training schedule.

Traer and Madhavan [29] studied the adoption of EP systems into UK clinical settings, especially into cancer networks, in a survey of cancer network lead pharmacists in the UK. They had a response rate of 63% and they found that 32% of respondents used chemotherapy EP systems and 8% used general EP systems. The authors noted that there was considerable national variance in the types of system available, and that more coordination was essential to ensure the development of quality systems.

Legal Requirements for EP Systems

An important area where the requirements of the state have an impact on EP systems is concerning the legal framework for prescribing. Many countries have laws restricting the right to prescribe, supply and personally administer medicines to certain professional groups, in order to safeguard the public and also to regulate the costs and the supply chain for medicines. As it is beyond the scope of this book to provide a full review of legal provisions around the world, and their implications for electronic prescribing systems, this section will be restricted an overview of the legal framework for prescribing in the UK, in order to illustrate some of the underlying issues for EP system designers.

The prescription, supply and administration of medicines in the UK is primarily regulated by the Medicines Act 1968, and its dependent legislation. The UK law defines Prescription Only Medicines (POMs) as those medicines where a legally valid prescription from a clinician is required before the medicine can be supplied to a patient for self-administration. However, in the UK, any medicine – including over the counter (OTC) medicines, and unlicensed medicines – may be prescribed (subject to any specific local restrictions). Consequently, when configuring drug datasets, implementers should not make the legal category of a medicine alone a condition for prescribability.

There is a provision in the law indicating that a medicine written on a hospital chart for administration by a nurse to a hospital inpatient is, in fact, an "order to administer" a medicine, rather than a prescription. Consequently, electronic medicine orders for outpatient and discharge supply legally constitute prescriptions, whereas electronic medicine orders for inpatients are orders for administration, which do not, in fact, need to conform fully to prescription regulations. Nevertheless, it has been regarded as good practice for all medicine orders generated in hospitals to comply with the legal requirements.

A legal prescription in the UK has the following attributes:

(a) It must be legible ("written in ink or otherwise so as to be indelible").
(b) It must be dated.
(c) It must include the name and address of the patient, and their age if under 12.
(d) It must be signed in ink by the prescriber.

The legal requirements for a prescription should be considered in the design of the dispensing screens of an EP system. It should be noted that provision (d) has hindered the use of UK hospital EP systems in the past, in that electronic outpatient and discharge prescriptions needed to be signed by hand to validate them. However, recently, UK law has been changed to enable a prescription to be validated with an advanced electronic signature [30]. Advanced electronic signatures are being used to support the community based Electronic Prescription Service in England [31] and would be useful for supporting hospital outpatient prescribing.

In the UK, some medicines are subject to specific controls under the Misuse of Drugs Act, 1971, and subsequent measures. These are known as Controlled Drugs (CDs), and are primarily medicines with an abuse potential, for example, opiates and stimulants. With these medicines, the following requirements apply in addition:

(a) It must specify the prescriber's address.
(b) It must include the dose and, for a preparation, the form and strength of the preparation.
(c) It must include the total quantity in words and figures.

Again, these data items must be included in the prescription profile or dispensing screen for CDs

In the UK, there is a requirement to maintain registers of the receipt and supply of CDs. In recent years, this requirement has enhanced to include the recording of:

(a) running balances
(b) the name of the supplying pharmacist, and
(c) the name of the person collecting the medicine.

These enhancements enable a fuller audit trail of the supply of controlled drugs to be established. In 2005, the England Misuse of Drugs Regulations were amended to allow the maintenance of electronic CD registers. In 2007, the England Department of Health issued guidance on the management of controlled drugs in hospitals, which included requirements for features of electronic CD registers [32]. There are a number of design features which need to be included in an electronic CD register:

- The author of each register entry must be identifiable.
- It must not be possible to amend entries after they have been made.
- All entries should be attributable to an individual.
- There must be an audit log of all register transactions.
- There must be an adequate back-up system.
- Systems must be in place to minimize the risk of unauthorized access to the register data.

Electronic CD registers are now being implemented in UK hospitals.[6] As well as the obvious benefit of preventing written transcription errors, electronic CD registers have been shown to reduce the time taken for register entries to be made, and enforce access control for individuals authorized to issue CDs and to make register adjustments. The electronic CD register is likely to be part of the pharmacy system and enables the possibility of automated issue of CDs from a pharmacy robot, subject to the availability of the required storage module on the robot.

A significant proportion of medicines used in hospitals are for unlicensed, or "off label" use, where the manufacturer does not have regulatory approval to promote it for that use. Some cases, a licensed medicine is used for an unlicensed indication, or in a patient group where it doesn't have a license – the use of medicines licensed for adults in children is a common scenario. Alternatively, a completely unlicensed medicine is supplied by a manufacturer for a specific purpose, possibly for compassionate reasons. It should be noted that it is not illegal to prescribe unlicensed medicines, but that the prescriber, rather than the drug company, takes full responsibility for prescribing the drug. Consequently, it is desirable for EP systems to indicate clearly to a prescriber if a product is unlicensed.

EP Systems and Professional Liability

Medicine is one of the most highly regulated areas of professional practice and, with an increasingly litigation-conscious culture and a corresponding increase in defensive practice on the part of health professions, awareness of professional liability will increase in forthcoming years. As a general principle, each individual practitioner is legally responsible for his or her decisions and actions as a healthcare professional, and the use of electronic systems as prescribing, dispensing and decision support

---

[6] See, for example, McCrea [33].

tools does not detract from this. Indeed, software vendors should include a disclaimer in their documentation to the effect that electronic prescribing software is a tool and is not intended to replace the clinical judgement of the practitioner.

However, while clinical users must still use their clinical judgement when prescribing electronically, they need to have sufficient confidence in the software to be able to use it routinely in a busy clinical environment. This confidence comes from rigorous testing of system configuration and software operations, prior to live use of the software, and detailed documentation of the pre-implementation configuration and testing of the software. This is called the "due diligence" process – so called because, if the healthcare provider were taken to court as a result of an error facilitated by the software, they would use the testing and acceptance documentation for their defence, to show that, in legal terms, they had "exercized due diligence" in assessing the risks of implementing the software. The UK medicines and devices regulator, the Medicines and Healthcare Regulatory Agency (MHRA), considers EP systems and other automated systems as medical devices if they use algorithms whose operation is not transparent to the end user.

It is possible that an EP system could facilitate a critical incident as a result of the operation of the software or its configuration. In this situation, the software vendor may be liable along with the practitioner and the healthcare provider. It is essential then that software vendors utilize appropriate clinical expertise when designing an EP system, that they have appropriate arrangements in place for the provision of drug data for their EP system (see Chap. 5), and that they ensure that appropriate due diligence documentation is generated, as part of the implementation project management.

However, following a recent review of prescribing errors by the UK General Medical Council [34], it has been suggested that professional regulators may in future mandate the use of electronic systems by practitioners where available in order to reduce human error rates with prescribing practice [11].

Confidentiality and Consent

Health professionals and health providers who hold personal information about their patients and clients have a duty of confidence to the people about whom the information is held (the subjects of the information). This is well-established in English case law, the English Data Protection Act and also European law and Federal Law in the US. In addition, there is an ethical obligation to maintain professional standards of confidentiality for many health professions.

The data protection principles are that that information given or received in confidence for one purpose may not be used for another purpose, or disclosed to a third party without the subject's consent. The duty of confidence continues after the death of the subject, and after a professional has ceased professional practice.

The use of EP systems, which contain prescription and medicines-related information about patients, is, of course, subject to the recognized confidentiality requirements. In 1997, the Caldicott Committee reported on issues relating to security and confidentiality of patient information [35] in the UK, and indicated that patient-based information systems used in the NHS should be designed in a secure way, with *privacy-enhancing technologies* incorporated within the application structure. These requirements have more recently been incorporated in the England CfH information governance agenda for healthcare professions [36].

There are a number of guiding principles for safeguarding confidentiality of patient information in electronic systems:

(a) System databases should have appropriate internal security, and patient data should be anonymized within them.
(b) Consideration should be given to appropriate encryption when data are transferred outside the system.
(c) A user's level of access should be appropriate to their role.
(d) A system should indicate in some way that the user is viewing confidential information
(e) Identifiable information relating to UK patients should not be processed outside of the UK.

A particular issue that has been debated is the way in which especially sensitive personal information is stored on an electronic system – for example, information on a person's HIV infection status, or a record of their treatment at sexually transmitted diseases (STD) clinic. While it is necessary for this information to be recorded electronically and, as far as possible, taken into account by decision support functions, consideration should be given limiting access to that information, or providing some form of "sealed envelope" functionality to prevent the information being viewed freely by all users.

Related to the matter of confidentiality is the issue of a patient's consent to having their information stored on an EP system. In many instances, a patient's consent is implied when a medication history is taken from a general practitioner's letter; the assumption is that the patient agreed to the referral. Indeed, in many scenarios, it has to be assumed that consent is implied; if consent had to be obtained explicitly at every stage of the patient care process, the work of a healthcare provider would soon become unmanageable. However, in situations where information – for example, a prescribing history – is elicited from a patient, or when other information is obtained from the patient (such as the medicines review scenario described in Chap. 6), with the intention of putting the information on the EP system, then explicit consent should be obtained from the patient to store the data for a nominated purpose. This is consistent with the requirements of the UK data protection legislation.

Ethical Issues

As EP systems will be operated by healthcare professionals, the ethical principles followed by healthcare professionals (which are made explicit in the codes of ethics published by professional bodies), are of significance when considering the use of EP systems. It is well established in many legal systems that a health professional has a "<u>duty of care</u>" for their patients – that the healthcare professional will ensure that the patient is treated according to recognized <u>best practice</u>, has the most appropriate treatment for their illness, and that the patient's interests are best served. For this reason, healthcare professionals will want to be assured that an EP system will optimize the therapeutic decision-making process for the patient, will reduce any known risks associated with the prescribing process, and will ensure that confidential patient information is stored and retrieved in a reliable and secure manner.

Furthermore, if an EP system has any specific operational shortcomings, either due to software bugs or data configuration issues, then health professionals will want these issues to be rectified by the software vendor, in the interests of the healthcare provider and the patient population. However, this may bring them into conflict with software vendors, whose prime motivations are commercial and political, and who may not wish to allocate resource to resolve outstanding issues as there is no extra revenue for doing so. In particular, this may lead to conflicts of interest for health professionals who are employed by software vendors.

<u>Resource allocation</u> is an ongoing issue in modern healthcare providers, due to increased burdens of healthcare requirements, and a finite budget to meet those requirements. While resource allocation is a reality for health professionals, they may be concerned at the potential for EP systems to impose government restrictions on prescribing practice, or to apply such restrictions in an unrealistic manner, without regard to the professional's <u>clinical judgment</u>.

Conclusion

EP systems have been implemented successfully in some healthcare economies and have been associated with various clinical and organisational benefits. Furthermore, there is a huge potential for greater adoption of EP systems, and introduction of progressively more complex functionality. However, the design, implementation and operation of EP systems necessarily takes place in a world where there are complex interactions of sociopolitical, psychological, legal and technical factors, affecting EP implementation. System designers need to bear in mind that EP systems are "<u>sociotechnical systems</u>", where both the system and the people using it influence the benefits and outcomes of system use, and also any legal, professional and ethical issues associated with system use. Given the potential impact of EP systems on a wide range of stakeholders, these issues should be explored in greater detail, both as part of multidisciplinary EP implementation projects, and also by specific experts in the issues involved.

References

1. Barbarito F. Regional service card health and social care information system. Presented at opportunities in e-Health. London; 2006.
2. Sjoborg B, Backstrom T, et al. Design and implementation of a point-of-care computerised system for drug therapy in Stockholm metropolitan health region – bridging the gap between knowledge and practice. Int J Med Inform. 2007;76:497–506.
3. Bell DS, Friedman MA. E-prescribing and the medicare modernisation act of 2003. Health Aff. 2005;24:1159–69.
4. NHS Connecting for Health. Electronic prescribing in hospitals: challenges & lessons learnt. 2009. http://www.connectingforhealth.nhs.uk/systemsandservices/eprescribing. p. 10–11. Accessed in October 2011.
5. NHS Connecting for Health. Electronic prescribing in hospitals: challenges & lessons learnt. 2009. http://www.connectingforhealth.nhs.uk/systemsandservices/eprescribing. p. 9.
6. Shane R. Computerized physician order entry: challenges and opportunities. Am J Health Syst Pharm. 2002;59:286–8. Accessed in October 2011.
7. Jones ML. Information management for health professions. Albany: Delmar, NY, USA; 1996. p. 64–5.
8. Goundrey-Smith SJ. Electronic prescribing – experience in the UK and system design issues. Pharm J. 2006;277:485–9.
9. Bonnabry P, Despont-Gros C, et al. A risk analysis method to evaluate the impact of a computerized provider order entry system on patient safety. J Am Med Inform Assoc. 2008;15:453–60.
10. Bates DW, Gawande AA. Improving safety with information technology. N Engl J Med. 2003;248:2526–34.
11. Goundrey-Smith SJ. Has electronic prescribing reached its tipping point? National Health Service Executive. 2010. http://www.bj-hc.co.uk/views/views-news-detail.html?news=1717&lang=en&feed=125. p. 70–71.
12. Koppel R, Metlay JD, et al. Role of computerized physician order entry systems in facilitating medication errors. J Am Med Assoc. 2005;293:1197–203.
13. Rogers EM. Diffusions of innovation. 5th ed. New York: Free Press; 2005. p. 22.
14. Goundrey-Smith SJ. Electronic prescribing – technology designed for the healthcare setting. Pharm J. 2007;278:677–8, 683.
15. Coiera E. Guide to health informatics. 2nd ed. London: Arnold; 2003. p. 202–22.
16. Hammond B. Electronic prescribing: developing the solution. Hosp Pharm. 2007;14:221–2, 224.
17. Sanghani P. Hospitals must embrace electronic prescribing. Pharm J. 2011;286:331.
18. Barber N. Electronic prescribing – safer, faster, better? J Health Serv Res Policy. 2010;15 Suppl 1:64–7.
19. Pheby D, Etherington DJ. Improving the comparability of cancer registry treatment data and proposals for a new national minimum dataset. J Public Health Med. 1994;16:331–40.
20. NHS Connecting for Health. Electronic prescribing in hospitals: challenges & lessons learnt. 2009. http://www.connectingforhealth.nhs.uk\systemsandservices\eprescribing. Accessed in October 2011.
21. Swanson D. Electronic prescribing – "I wannit and I wannit now" hosp. Pharm J. 2007;14:210.
22. Fincham J. E-prescribing – the electronic tranformation of medicine. Sudbury: Jones & Bartlett; 2009.
23. Van Ornum M. Electronic prescribing: a safety and implementation guide. Sudbury: Jones & Bartlett; 2009.
24. Abdel Qader DH, Cantrill JA, Tully MP. Satisfaction predictors and attitudes towards electronic prescribing systems in three UK hospitals. Pharm World Sci. 2010;32:581–93.
25. Steinschaden T, Petersson G, Astrand B. Physicians' attitudes towards E-prescribing: a comparative web survey in Austria and Sweden. Inform Prim Care. 2009;17:241–8.
26. Hellstrom L, Waern K, Montelius E, Rydberg T, Petersson G. Physicians' attitudes to E-prescribing: evaluation of a Swedish full-scale implementation. BMC Med Inform Decis Mak. 2009;9:37.

27. Tan WS, Phang JS, Tan LK. Evaluating user satisfaction with an electronic prescription system in a primary care group. Ann Acad Med Singapore. 2009;38:494–7.
28. Mehta R, Onatade R. Experience of electronic prescribing in UK hospitals: a perspective from pharmacy staff. Pharm J. 2008;281:79–82.
29. Traer E, Madhavan K. Electronic prescribing and transfer/discharge summaries: a survey of UK cancer networks. Pharm J. 2010;284:453–4.
30. Medicines, ethics & practice. 35th ed. Royal Pharmaceutical Society. London; 2011. p. 21.
31. NHS Connecting for Health. EPS release 2: business process guidance for initial implementers. 2009. p. 74–9. http://www.connectingforhealth.nhs.uk/systemsandservices/eps/library/comms/release2/bpg/release2guide.pdf Accessed in October 2011.
32. Safer management of controlled drugs – a guide to good practice in secondary care (England). England Department of Health. 2007. p. 58. http://www.dh.gov.uk/prod_consum_dh/groups/dh_digitalassets/documents/digitalasset/dh_079591.pdf Accessed in October 2011.
33. McCrea G. Presented at guild of healthcare pharmacists/UK clinical pharmacy association information technology interest group seminar. 2011. http://www.ghp.org.uk/ContentFiles/ghpitig11f.pps. Accessed in October 2011.
34. General Medical Council. An in-depth investigation into causes of prescribing errors by foundation trainees in relation to their medical education – EQUIP study; 2009. http://www.gmc-uk.org/FINAL_Report_prevalence_and_causes_of_prescribing_errors.pdf_28935150.pdf.
35. Caldicott Committee. Report on the review of patient identifiable information. London: Department of Health; 1997.
36. Goundrey-Smith SJ. Ensure your IT systems are compliant by March. Pharm J. 2011;286:40.

Chapter 2
History and Context of Electronic Prescribing in the US and UK

The Development of Information Technology in Healthcare

With the advent of solid state technology, where for the first time it was possible to build computers that were powerful enough to handle large volumes of data with optimal speed, but small enough to be of practical use in a working environment, organizations began to see the potential of computer-based systems to replace paper records of different sorts.

Within healthcare, the first major area of IT application was the use of electronic systems to facilitate the collection, storage and dissemination of discrete, patient-related data (either numeric or coded with a recognized coding methodology) as a solution to specific healthcare activities. Consequently, over the last 20 years, the most well-developed IT applications in secondary care have been (a) pathology systems, for the management of test results, and (b) pharmacy systems, for the labeling of dispensed items and for pharmacy stock control. Systems such as these were relatively straightforward to implement, as they had their hub in one particular department of the hospital (and this department therefore had control over the implementation), the benefits of such systems were substantial in comparison to the potential risks, and they presented no special problems concerning database and communications technology. Subsequent IT applications in secondary care included whole-hospital systems such as patient administration systems (PAS) and order communications, dealing with the messaging of orders in the broadest sense (e.g. radiology orders as well as pathology and pharmacy orders).

Correspondingly, in primary care, GP systems have been in use since the mid 1980s and, in recent years, have become quite elaborate, in terms of the functionality they offer. As well as the ability to store clinical notes (usually with a problem/note hierarchy) and generate prescriptions, these systems are able to provide prescription pricing information, detailed medical information from reference sources such as the British National Formulary (BNF) or the Physicians Desk Reference, pathology order management and items of service/billing and claim management.

S. Goundrey-Smith, *Principles of Electronic Prescribing*, Health Informatics, 25
DOI 10.1007/978-1-4471-4045-0_2, © Springer-Verlag London 2012

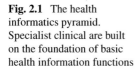

Fig. 2.1 The health informatics pyramid. Specialist clinical are built on the foundation of basic health information functions

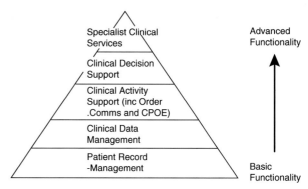

However, the issue facing all users of healthcare systems is that of their intraoperability. This has particularly been an issue in secondary care where a hospital has, historically, had a number of computer systems – a <u>PAS</u>, a <u>pathology system</u>, a <u>pharmacy system</u>, a <u>radiology system</u> – offering reliable functionality, but operating in parallel, in a "silo" fashion, with no connectivity between them. This presents a number of problems – (a) duplication of effort in the design and configuration of functions that may be common to all systems (e.g. patient selection functions), (b) duplication of staff effort in data entry onto the systems, (c) introduction of risk due to all elements of a patient record not being visible to a user through a single system. As discussed previously, one of the key goals of <u>regional and national healthcare IT programs</u> is systems <u>integration</u>, in order to eradicate these problems. Nevertheless, a higher level of <u>intraoperability</u>, supported by appropriate <u>coding methodologies</u>, and a willingness of all <u>stakeholders</u> to work towards an integrated system are essential to realize this goal.

In any case, aside from the issues of <u>silo development</u> and <u>intraoperability</u>, there are some areas of <u>secondary care</u> that have not as yet been adequately catered for with IT applications. These are primarily clinical applications, most notably the so-called <u>"electronic patient record" (EPR)</u> and the broader term <u>"electronic health record" (EHR)</u>. These areas have not been so well developed possibly because of (a) the complexity of algorithms required to perform the required clinical decision support on EPR data; (b) the lack of expertise available for the design of these systems by IT vendors, and (c) the reliance of such systems on the availability of adequate technology for handling images (X-rays, MRI scans, CAT scans etc.). One of the clinical applications still in its infancy is electronic prescribing.

If hospital information services can be illustrated as a pyramid, EP systems constitute the pinnacle of the pyramid, and are built on the foundation of other more basic functionality (see Fig. 2.1).

Development of EP Systems in the United States

Much of the available published information on EP implementations originates from the United States. Electronic systems for medicine prescribing and administration have been adopted more widely in the US, possibly due to (a) the need for costing of medication administration, in an insurance-based health system, and (b) the need for risk management to reduce clinical risk to a minimum, and to optimize audit trails in a highly litigious society. As a consequence, there are many proprietary EP, or CPOE, systems available in the United States.

In the late 1990s, US Government Agencies increasingly began to recognize the potential for electronic prescribing systems to reduce clinical risk in busy hospitals.

In 1999 and 2001, the US Institute of Medicine (IOM) produced two well-publicized reports [1, 2], which looked at how technology could be used to support and improve patient safety. The 2001 report, *Crossing the Quality Chasm*, recommended that all stakeholders – providers, purchasers, clinicians and patients – collaborate in the redesign of healthcare processes, towards the goals of evidence-based medicine, knowledge sharing and patient empowerment [3].

Furthermore, in 2000, the commercial sector made a much-publicized call for an improvement to patient safety by the use of electronic systems. The Leapfrog Group – a coalition of major US companies, the Fortune 500 companies – have identified CPOE as one of the three changes that would most improve safety [4]. It is likely that many senior managers in the commercial sector see safety issues as a major cause of litigation and potential source of financial cost.

In the opening years of the twenty-first century, the US government began to make capital funding available for the implementation of new EP systems. For example, in 2001, the US Senate tabled the Medication Errors Reduction Act, to create a $1 billion federal grant program to help healthcare providers purchase EP systems. Also, in 2003, the House of Representatives passed the Patient Safety Improvement Act, which aimed to provide $50 million in grants over a 2-year period to organizations implementing information technology to improve patient safety [5].

Subsequently, one of the key drivers for functional development of existing EP systems was the Medicare Modernization Act (MMA) 2003, which recognized the capacity of electronic systems to produce efficiencies in risk reduction and cost savings in the management of chronic diseases [6]. The Act required that Part D Medicare plans should support an "electronic prescription program" should a healthcare provider choose to use one. In the Act, there was also permission for third party organizations to offset costs of implementation of EP systems by healthcare providers.

Specifically, the Act required the US Government Department of Health and Human Services to facilitate standards of interoperability in different functional areas, which are compatible with, and which build upon, existing standards. These include:

(a) ANSI ASC X12N 270/271 – to deal with eligibility and benefits enquires and responses between prescribers and insurance payers.
(b) National Council for Prescription Drug Programs (NCPDP) SCRIPT 5.1 – to deal with the majority of transactions between prescribers and dispensers, and
(c) NCPDP Telecommunication Standard 5.1 – to deal with eligibility and benefits enquires and responses between dispensers and insurance payers.

It is well recognized that commercial EP systems in the US vary in the level of advanced functionality they provide, in terms of decision support, and it has been suggested that there should be further legislation to incentivize the standardization of these advanced functions.

In the US, <u>decision support</u> applications have been used by clinicians at the point of prescribing for many years, and have been extensively evaluated in the medical literature – major reviews of the available studies were published in 1994 [7], and 1998 [8]. However, there was little published information on quantitative analysis of comprehensive EP systems until the late 1990s.

The most notable center for EP use in the US is the Brigham and Women's Hospital, Boston [9–11]. The Brigham and Women's CPOE functionality was developed in the early 1990s as part of an in-house information system, the Brigham Integrated Computing System, which was designed to manage all aspects of the hospital's administrative and clinical processes. The initial system included <u>formulary prescribing</u> menus, default doses/dose selection, display of relevant laboratory results and limited <u>sensitivity checking</u>, <u>drug interaction checking</u> and <u>laboratory test interaction checking</u>. Further checking functions were added in an upgrade to the system in 1996.

Another early implementation of CPOE was the system at the Wishard Memorial Hospital, Indianapolis, Indiana [12], which was implemented in the late 1980s, and documented in a study published in 1993. This system consisted of the Regenstrief Medical Records System mounted on a series of networked PCs through the wards and <u>emergency department</u> of the hospital. This system enabled electronic ordering and decision support on each ward and electronic transmission of orders to the pharmacies.

There have been published studies of other EP implementations in the US. Spencer et al. [13] describe the implementation of the Siemens Medical Solutions CPOE System at the University of North Carolina (UNC) Hospitals in 2002. The system was initially piloted on one general medicine floor at the hospitals in 2002 and was the further rolled out to a second medical floor, and a step-down critical care unit in 2003. The implementation was then studied by analysis of medication errors generated between February 2002 and May 2003.

Mekhjian and colleagues [14] have published their analysis of the implementation of an EP system at an academic medical center. They found that major process changes following the implementation of an advanced CPOE system did not adversely affect <u>hospital stay time</u> or <u>hospital stay cost</u>, but had a beneficial effect on turnaround times for <u>medicine supply</u> and <u>pathology test reporting</u> and <u>radiology test reporting</u>.

Koppel et al. [15] describe the operation of a commercial EP system (TDS) at the University of Pennsylvania between 1997 and 2004, and, in particular, a qualitative and quantitative analysis of system use, conducted during 2002–2003.

Recently, Stone et al. [16] implemented CPOE in a multi-specialty surgery facility at the Mayor Clinic, Phoenix, Arizona. They found that the system led to efficiency benefits and an initial risk reduction in the first 6 months after implementation, but they found that further system refinements would be required to give sustained patient safety improvements.

The US Health Information Technology for Economic and Clinical Health Act 2009 has led to increased adoption of electronic health records, by introducing the "meaningful use" criteria, which mandate the use of CPOE [17]. This has led to the growing adoption of EP systems in community and ambulatory settings in the US, which has been shown to reduce the dispensing error rate, compared with paper prescriptions [18].

Studies of US EP implementations have showed a number of benefits of EP, notably: (a) reduction in medication error rate; (b) a reduction in transcription error rate (as would be expected); (c) a reduction in medicine supply turn-around times (due to electronic communication between the ward and the pharmacy); (d) a modest reduction in hospital stay time, and (e) an improvement in radiology test reporting and laboratory test reporting times (due to fully electronic communication processes). However, these benefits may not be realizable to the same extent in other health economies due to differences in health service structure, clinical practice and medicine costing and reimbursement.

Two of the US studies, however, highlight the potential for EP systems to generate, or facilitate new types of medication error, an issue that will be examined in greater detail in a subsequent chapter.

Development of EP Systems in the United Kingdom

The adoption of EP systems in the UK has been equally slow. In early 2007, it was reported that only three hospitals in England (the Wirral Hospitals, Burton on Trent and Winchester) had whole-hospital electronic prescribing systems [19]. This is broadly consistent with a survey of 188 hospitals conducted in the UK in 2000 [20], indicating that, at the time, 89.4% of hospitals surveyed had no EP system, 11% had an EP system but only 2% of hospitals had full electronic prescribing facilities. This suggests that the uptake of EP systems in UK centers has been slow over the past 10 years. The likely scenario is that the English Connecting for Health IT program slowed down local EP innovation, as reported in Chap. 1 [21]. In any case, the difficulties associated with EP implementations, due to commercial and organizational factors have been commented on in the literature [22, 23].

UK hospitals have a good track-record of technology innovation over the past 20 or 30 years. Enterprise-wide patient administration systems (PAS) have become commonplace. Pharmacy systems in the UK came into routine use in the mid 1980s, following a change in the law requiring labels to be in typeface rather than handwritten. Pathology systems for test result processing and reporting have also been in use since the 1980s. However, as mentioned previously, these systems have largely developed in a separate "silo" fashion, as individual departmental systems. Consequently, one of the most significant tasks in any new healthcare software implementation is not necessarily establishing the technical platform (networks and servers), or configuring the software, but designing and testing the interfaces required between the new application and other hospital systems. A typical example of such an interface would be between, for example, a pathology system or pharmacy system and a hospital PAS, to provide a feed of patient demographic data to the departmental system. The use of "service oriented architecture" has the potential to surmount intraoperability issues within healthcare provider organizations. The business process rationale for using a service-oriented architecture will be discussed in Chap. 3.

The UK centers with the longest history of EP innovation are the Wirral Hospitals, in Cheshire, England, and the Burton Hospitals, Burton on Trent, Staffordshire, England.

The Wirral Hospitals began implementing their EP service as part of an integrated hospital information system (HIS) in 1992, and by 2002, they had achieved Level 4 electronic patient record (EPR) status [24]. The Wirral Hospitals subsequently installed an automated dispensing system (pharmacy robot) in 2001.

The Burton on Trent Trust have also been working with electronic medicines management systems since 1992 [25]. Queen's Hospital, Burton, had a modular Meditech HISS (hospital information support system) already in place, and implemented the pharmacy module of the Meditech system in 1992. In 1995, the Trust was selected by the then NHS Information Management Group to be one of two sites to participate in the Electronic Patient Record (EPR) program. The chief criteria for this was that the Trust was already operating an integrated HISS and had commitment from all the major stakeholders in the implementation process – clinicians, hospital management and suppliers. The EPR program included electronic prescribing as one its sub-projects and, when the EPR program was complete in December 1996, three pilot wards in the elderly care directorate were using the EP system. The system was subsequently extended to two further care of the elderly wards, the admissions unit and the ophthalmology ward. The EP system at Burton offered integration with the hospital EPR system, easy to use medicine look-up lists and clear display of patient medication records, modeled on the Trust's standard treatment card. The area that provided some difficulties for the team at Burton was the implementation of an appropriate level of decision support within the system. This is an important issue in EP design and will be discussed in a subsequent chapter.

Case Study 1: The Winchester & Eastleigh NHS Trust
Two Generations of Electronic Prescribing
The Winchester & Eastleigh NHS Trust, in the south of England, was the first hospital to implement electronic prescribing in the UK, and has been working with electronic prescribing functionality for over 20 years. In the mid 1980s, as a result of a government initiative, the Winchester Trust received some regional funding to enable them to deploy advanced IT within the hospital. The Trust purchased the American TDS Hospital Information System (HIS), and invested time and resources to configure the system to a UK context.

The Trust Board took a strong line in implementing the technology at a time when there was considerably less experience with IT applications in acute clinical environments. The implementation project was managed by the IM&T department and various pharmacy and nursing personnel were seconded to the project as domain analysts. In addition, in-house analysts and trainers were provided by TDS. A programme of acceptance testing was conducted whereby users changed roles (prescribers became pharmacy users and vice versa etc.), prior to installation.

The system was piloted on surgical wards, and rolled out across the whole hospital during 1989–1990. Problems with the implementation of the software centred around three areas (a) certain aspects of the EP software – for example, non-scheduled intravenous fluid ordering did not function to suit working practices in the UK, and were complicated (b) hardware support for the mainframe had to be negotiated for 24/7 coverage instead of the usual 9–5 business hours and (c) staff attitudes to the system at a time when computers were an unknown to most staff, and perhaps something to be worried about.

When launched, the system consisted of a mainframe with three static terminals on each 30 bed ward (two terminals on smaller wards) and five terminals in the pharmacy, all connected by a token ring network. As technologies improved, mobile workstations were introduced and now the system operates with three mobile workstations on each ward as well as the static ones. The system is now supported by an Ethernet network.

For some time after initial roll-out, the system was not wholly popular with some hospital staff, partly because of the changes that it entailed, and partly because of the change management process. However, clinicians soon began to see the advantages of an electronic system – especially when they left the Trust to work elsewhere, and had to return to paper-based systems. The system has enabled the expansion of clinical pharmacy services on the wards, has considerably improved the workflow in the dispensary, and has also increased the efficiency of the pharmacy emergency on call system.

Over the years, various methodologies have been employed to train new users. Initially the approach was didactic, with formal training sessions. However, the training now consists of a talk and demonstration by a trainer, with training exercises on a training data environment, and then ward-based follow-up. A one-to-one training program would be ideal but this would be impossible to implement, given the high turn-over of users.

Because of the increasing cost of support for the TDS system, together with the requirement at the time to adopt CfH (Cerner) functionality for other hospital systems, the Trust implemented the JAC Computer Services EP module (JAC Computer Services, Basildon, UK) in 2006, as the interim "next generation" EP system, and the TDS system prescribing module was decommissioned. The JAC EP system offers the advantage of an intuitive Windows-based system, medicines administration functionality that closely mimics the traditional drug chart, and which is therefore readily acceptable to all users, and third party data support from First DataBank Europe (FDBE) Ltd (Exeter, UK). The third party data platform is of particular importance because this enables the system to undertake comprehensive decision support on drug interactions, allergies and other clinical warnings. JAC send a monthly FDBE data update to Winchester.

With almost 20 years of EP experience in the Trust, electronic prescribing is now part of the culture at the Winchester and Eastleigh NHS Trust, and Trust personnel have built up considerable expertise in the practical use of EP

Systems. However, in 2012, the Winchester and Eastleigh NHS Trust is due to merge with the neighboring Basingstoke Trust and a decision will need to be made about how electronic prescribing will be supported across the new merged Trust. Possible future plans for system development include outpatient prescribing and IV fluid prescribing.

Fowlie et al. [26] conducted an analysis of prescribing errors and medicine administration errors at Ayr Hospital, Scotland, following the introduction of an electronic prescribing and medicines administration system (Pharmakon). The system was evaluated in a 36 bed orthopedic ward between February 1998 and July 1999. The authors compared rates of prescribing errors for inpatient and discharge prescriptions and rates of administration error for (a) the existing paper-based prescribing system, (b) electronic prescribing 1 month after implementation, and (c) electronic prescribing 12 months after implementation. They found that the electronic prescribing system led to a significant reduction in the prescribing error rate for inpatient prescriptions but, interestingly, not for discharge prescriptions, and that the system led to a significant reduction in medication administration errors. The impact these results on medication risk management will be discussed in detail in a later chapter.

Gray and Smith [27] reported on the implementation of an electronic prescribing system on surgical wards at Southmead Hospital, Bristol. Southmead Hospital, which is now part of the North Bristol NHS Trust, embarked on an EPR project in 1997 using the Sunrise Clinical Manager software, which subsequently became iSOFT's iClinical Manager (iCM).[1] This established electronic order communications in the hospital for pathology tests, radiology procedures and selected clinic referrals. In January 2001, Southmead Hospital embarked on a 2-year project to establish an electronic prescribing and electronic medicines administration system throughout the hospital, using the Sunrise/iCM system. However, during the course of the project, the scope was reviewed, for financial and strategic reasons, and the EP system was limited to pilot use in the surgical unit. The EP system was piloted between September and December 2002 on the surgical admissions ward, two general surgical wards and the associated theatres and recovery rooms.

The system had electronic drug administration functions and an interface with the Trust's pharmacy system. However, it did not have comprehensive decision support functions; sensitivity checking and duplicate therapy checking were available within the application but were not implemented, and no third party clinical rules engine was employed. The charting of anesthetics and fluids was not included on the system.

Since the completion of the Southmead pilot, other NHS Trusts have piloted the iCM product for electronic medicines management applications, using enhancements arising from the Southmead project. One such pilot was at Hope Hospital,

---

[1] iCM functionality was incorporated into the iSOFT integrated product, Lorenzo, which was developed for the English NHS Connecting for Health Project.

Salford [28], where an EPR project was launched using the Sunrise iCM software in 1999. The EPR system went live in mid 2000, and allowed storage of admission history and correspondence, electronic ordering of radiology tests, and electronic discharge summaries. Electronic discharge summaries have been a significant development in electronic medicines management in UK hospitals, and will be discussed in a later section of this chapter.

EP has been implemented at City Hospitals, Sunderland using Meditech software, as used at the Burton Hospitals [29]. In Sunderland, other modules of the Meditech software have been in use by pharmacists and nurses since 1992, but medical staff have had little experience of the system prior to the introduction of electronic prescribing and medicines administration. Consequently, adoption of the system by medical staff was therefore a major aspect of the change management required to roll out the EP system at Sunderland. EP functionality has been available at City Hospitals, Sunderland since 2002 [30].

In their review of the implementation process for EP, Foot and Taylor [29] noted a number of benefits with the system. These included: (a) a reduction in the overall prescribing process duration; (b) the ability of staff to access patient records from remote locations (leading to further time and logistical efficiencies), and (c) a clear audit trail of signatures for each prescription.

Case Study 2: Shrewsbury & Telford NHS Trust
The eSCRIPT Electronic Transcribing System
The Shrewsbury and Telford NHS Trust is an acute healthcare provider in Shropshire, UK, which has developed eSCRIPT, an electronic system which enables prescriptions transcribed from the wards to be fulfilled in the pharmacy. Because the prescription history is captured electronically, a patient medication record (PMR) and legible discharge documentation can be generated for each patient.

The eSCRIPT system was developed in-house at the Trust with a Crystal database platform, a custom-designed user interface and links with the PAS and bed management systems. The rationale for developing the system was to streamline the discharge process, produce legible discharge prescriptions and to support the work of ward-based clinical pharmacists. Work on the system was commenced in 1999, and it was initially piloted on a few wards (long-stay stroke/rehabilitation wards), before being rolled out across the hospital over a period of 18 months.

The system consists of a central server, networked with wireless workstations on the wards, mounted on Psion Netbook devices. The key benefit of the system is that it provides a PMR, supply record and discharge summary for a patient within the same system. The system is generally popular because (a) the initial design process was led by the users (a benefit of an in-house system) and, (b) key stakeholders (pharmacists, IM&T staff and clinical divisional leads) were engaged early on during the project.

While the system was tested at the outset using a variety of patient scenarios and use cases, a number of issues became apparent once the system became fully operational. These concerned the management of patient's own drugs (PODs) by the system, and the recording of POD use in long-term patients. Related to this was the development of an interface with the EDS pharmacy system, which is used by the Trust. So far, it has not been possible to produce a reliable interface, and it is still necessary to rekey information from eSCRIPT into the pharmacy system.

The system is administered by two senior pharmacists, and uses third party drug data from First DataBank Europe (FDBE) Ltd (Exeter, UK). FDBE send regular updates to the Trust, which are loaded onto the system by Trust IM&T staff, who then itemise any data changes for the attention of the system administrators. Based on FDBE data, the system provides decision support for drug interactions, sensitivities, drug-disease interactions, duplicate therapies and clinical trials management (trust customised table). The training of new users of the system is an in-use process consisting of a combination of desk-based initial training, together with shadowing experienced users.

The system was implemented with the view that, if the Connecting for Health (CfH) program did not deliver a timely EP solution, the eSCRIPT system could be expanded to become a thoroughgoing electronic prescribing and medicine administration system. The CfH program has now been discontinued, so the Shrewsbury & Telford NHS Trust now need to make a decision about how EP might be developed in the Trust. Expanding the eSCRIPT system as first envisaged would be a major program of work, but replacing the eSCRIPT system with a commercially-available EP system would also be an onerous task. Meanwhile, the eSCRIPT system is being maintained and managed on an ongoing basis.

An electronic prescribing system has been in use on a surgical ward at Charing Cross Hospital since 2003 [31] As well as the clinician interface, this system has a novel medicine administration system involving an electronic dispensing cabinet ("magic cupboard") and an electronic drug trolley on the ward, to facilitate accurate medicines administration. It is therefore a "closed loop" system.

The system was evaluated fully between 2003 and 2006 for risk management capacity, time requirements, user acceptability, stock control and audit trailing. The system has been shown to have a positive effect on the rates of both medicine prescribing errors and medicine administration errors.

Nightingale et al. [32] have evaluated a rules-based electronic prescribing system, which was designed for use with pen-based portable PCs and has been used on the renal unit at the Queen Elizabeth Medical Centre, Birmingham. In 1996, the renal unit at the Queen Elizabeth Hospital and the Wolfson Computer Laboratory embarked on a project to develop a rules-based prescribing system, with the intention of improving prescribing safety on the renal unit. The system developed was based on a Windows user interface and, as well as patient demographic data and prescribing history, the system handled data such as laboratory results, diagnosis, allergies and renal function calculations (Cockcroft Gault).

The system was introduced into the renal unit in January 1998, and a study of its use was conducted between October 1998 and August 1999. The system was used with 1,646 patients in this study, with a total of 87,789 prescriptions. The study found that, of these 87,789 orders, 58 prescriptions were disallowed for clinical reasons by the system – these were allergies and serious drug interactions. The authors concluded that the system made a positive impact on safe and effective prescribing on the renal unit.

The system, known as the Prescribing Information and Communications System (PICS), has now been rolled out across the University of Birmingham Hospitals [33]. The system roll out was completed in 2008, and it provides many benefits to the Trust, including prescribing decision support and the implementation of local and national clinical guidance.

Kings College Hospital, London, UK, [34] has implemented EP again using iSOFT's iCM system. The system was piloted in 2008, with a view to rolling the system out across the Trust in 18 months. Use of iCM meant that the EP and medicines administration system was integral to the electronic patient record. While the implementation process was a relatively complex one, because of the many configuration options with iCM, the end result was a system that was customized to the Trust's procedures.

The Freeman Hospital, Newcastle upon Tyne, UK [35] implemented the EP module of the enterprise-wide solution, Cerner Millennium, which was already installed in the Trust for PAS, accident & emergency (A&E), order communications and scheduling. EP functions included inpatient prescribing, discharge prescribing and pharmacy validation. Again, the system is highly configurable and the build process was laborious. However, the system went live in A&E in November 2009, and rolled out across all wards at the Freeman Hospital by April 2010.

In 2010, in a survey commissioned by the English Connecting for Health program, Cornford et al. [36] interviewed staff in 13 NHS Trusts and reviewed some of the major implementation issues and lessons learnt.

Development of EP Systems: A European Perspective

A survey of the use of electronic prescriptions in Europe, conducted in 2003 [37], indicated that automated solutions for electronic prescribing were not in widespread use in Europe and that the only two countries where electronic prescriptions were issued routinely were Denmark and Sweden. Pilot studies had taken place in the United Kingdom, and Germany had plans to implement electronic prescriptions. This study related primarily to electronic prescriptions in primary care and was concerned with the development of an EU-wide standard for dispensing and reimbursement of prescriptions. However, it is likely then that adoption of EP systems in secondary care in continental Europe has been equally slow.

There are few published reports of medicines management software applications used in hospitals in European countries. In a study of the implementation of hospital EP systems in Spain published in 2005 [38], responses from 47 Spanish hospitals were analyzed. Thirteen hospitals (27.7%) had EP systems and a further 15 (31.9%) were due to implement an EP system in the near future. Software used varied in its functionality but few of the applications implemented were able to be integrated with other systems to promote seamless pharmaceutical care. In a paper published in 2003 [39], Llopis Salvia and colleagues described the implementation of an EP system at the Hospital de la Ribera at Alzira, Valencia, Spain. The system offered integration with the whole hospital information system, computerized physician order entry and integration with pharmaceutical care activities.

Nielsen and Dybwik [40] have described the use of <u>decision support</u> software in <u>Norway</u> to alert <u>intensive care unit</u> clinicians to <u>drug interactions</u>. They used the internet based decision support system, <u>DRUID</u> (www.druid.uio.no) to evaluate drug interactions of drugs prescribed for patients during the first 24 h of their intensive care stay. Using the system, they identified 274 potential drug interactions in 110 patients. However, while just over half of the interactions required extra precautions to be taken (e.g. dose reduction), there were very few serious interactions noted.

There are also a number of reports evaluating systems implemented in Switzerland [41], Belgium [42] and the Netherlands [43, 44].

Development of EP Systems: An Australian Perspective

Computerized systems to support prescribing are in use in Australia in both primary and secondary care. Research has been conducted in Australian centers on clinical decision support [45–47], and workflow analysis [48] relating to the hospital prescribing process, but there have been no studies (quantitative or qualitative) of actual EP implementations in Australia.

Electronic Discharge Summaries

One of the most beneficial features of the Salford (UK) implementation [49] was the introduction of <u>immediate discharge summaries (IDS)</u>. These were piloted in medical and care of the elderly wards in mid 2001, and rolled out to the whole hospital in 2002. This function enabled clinicians to assemble an <u>electronic discharge summary</u> for each patient, including drug ordering from picklists or pre-defined orders.

The rationale for the IDS function was to streamline the hospital <u>discharge</u> process, which is a significant issue in the UK context. If the process for patient discharge is inefficient then not only is quality of care reduced and patient/healthcare professional morale affected, but bed management in the hospital becomes difficult, and this has far-reaching implications for service planning and development. Another significant issue with the hospital discharge process is that, with the traditional consultant's letter, it takes some time for a patient's care plan – and current medication schedule – to be sent to the patient's GP. The quadruplicate discharge forms introduced recently have been a considerable improvement, but these can be – and often are – mislaid by patients and hospital staff. Electronic communication of hospital discharge information from secondary care to primary care constitutes a critical factor in addressing some of the logistical and communication issues associated with a patient's discharge from hospital.

In recent years, while UK hospitals have been waiting for a national EP solution from NHS Connecting for Health, many UK hospitals have sought to develop interim electronic solutions for managing the discharge process, and therefore addressing a key issue for many hospitals. Some of these solutions have been implemented in a stand-alone fashion, others as a conscious step towards a full EP solution.

Two examples of UK electronic discharge systems are the eDischarge system at the Southampton Hospitals, UK, and the electronic transfer of care system at the Princess of Wales Hospital, Bridgend, Wales, UK. At Southampton [50], an e-discharge module was implemented as part of the Ascribe pharmacy management system. The system was piloted in the acute medical unit (AMU) in 2007. Based on this pilot, a second version of the software was launched on the medicine and care of the elderly wards and subsequently rolled out across the Trust. The system provides a direct transfer of discharge information to 30–40 GP surgeries in the locality, and a range of clinical and financial audit functions for hospital users. At the Princess of Wales Hospital, Bridgend [51], an electronic transfer of care system was developed in house to ensure that electronic information on a patient's medicines and care plan was generated and distributed to GPs in a timely manner. The system enabled discharge information to be available to primary care clinicians on the day of discharge for 96% of patients, a considerable improvement on previous paper-based systems.

Kirby et al. [52] conducted a case-control study of 102 patients processed by the electronic discharge system installed at King's Mill Hospital, Derbyshire, UK. They found a dramatic reduction in the time taken to generate a discharge summary with the electronic system, in comparison with the traditional paper-based discharge process (from a mean time of 80 days, to a mean time of 0 days ($p < 0.0001$)).

Work has also been done on the development of a common electronic discharge tool for hospitals throughout Wales, UK, using the Welsh Clinical Portal [53]. The system provides a common drug database and dose syntax (to support communication of prescribed doses) based on the dm+d medicines terminology (see Chap. 5). At the time of writing (early 2012), this system is about to be piloted in Cardiff & Vale Health Board.

Integration of EP Systems with Pharmacy Systems

As mentioned previously, the use of pharmacy systems became widespread in UK hospitals from the mid 1980s. The core functionalities of pharmacy computer systems were initially (a) to provide a legible label for each medicine, ensuring that all relevant information is displayed, according to legal and best practice requirements; (b) to maintain a record of the medicines issued to a patient, and the label instructions for each issue, and (c) to maintain a pharmacy stock control record of each pharmaceutical product, so that drug usage could be monitored.

However, as systems have developed, they have inevitably become more sophisticated. Many systems now have complex stock control algorithms to take into account <u>contract purchasing</u> and <u>cost-center billing</u>. They have modules for specialist manufacturing, such as <u>total parenteral nutrition</u>, <u>chemotherapy</u> and <u>central intravenous additives services (CIVAS)</u>. Many have interfaces with hand-held terminals to enable real-time stock control by <u>pharmacy support staff</u> on wards.

Due to their increasing sophistication, the scope of <u>pharmacy systems</u> in the UK has been expanding since 2000. There has previously been an initiative to link pharmacy system reporting to the central NHS supply chain project, under the auspices of the <u>NHS Purchasing and Supplies Agency (PASA)</u>. There is a need to link pharmacy systems with <u>pharmaceutical wholesaler systems</u> to enable <u>e-procurement</u>.

In response to the increasing adoption of automated dispensing systems (<u>pharmacy robots</u>), pharmacy systems need to be interfaced to an automated dispensing system in many hospital pharmacies in the UK. Furthermore, due to their expertise in software for managing <u>medicines information</u>, the key pharmacy system providers in the UK, JAC Systems and Ascribe, have been developing electronic prescribing modules for use in conjunction with their pharmacy systems. The most established example of this is the use of the JAC Systems EP module at the Royal Hampshire County Hospital, Winchester, UK. In 2006, the existing HIS prescribing functionality, which had been originally installed in 1989, was replaced by a second generation EP system from JAC. Thus, in the UK, despite the establishment of a national IT program, some healthcare providers are have implemented EP systems as an extension of their hospital pharmacy system, rather than as a module of a wider EPR system.

This distinction is worth noting because, while there is a need to link an EP system with a pharmacy system, many implementers stress the distinction between an EP system and a pharmacy system. An EP system is concerned with the effective and safe prescribing of medicines to a patient, whereas a pharmacy system is concerned with the accurate <u>stock-control</u>, assembly and <u>labeling</u> of medicinal products. In essence, an EP system is patient-centered, whereas a pharmacy system will be product-centered – although some commentators will argue that all medicines management related IT should be patient centered. The interface between an EP system and a pharmacy system therefore needs to provide an appropriate link between the distinctive functions of the system, so that these functions are not, in any way, duplicated in both systems. The reason why the relationship between a prescribing system and a pharmacy system should be carefully considered is because some IT vendors, particularly those with little prescribing or pharmacy <u>domain expertise</u> in house, tend to view medication functionality as a homogenous whole, and do not recognize the detailed design issues that have to be addressed to provide suitably comprehensive functionality.

In 2001, the <u>UK Audit Commission</u> published its report entitled "<u>A Spoonful of Sugar – Medicines Management in UK Hospitals</u>" [54]. This report looked at the "re-engineering" of healthcare <u>business processes</u> in UK hospitals, and in particular, highlighted the potential of automated dispensing systems (<u>pharmacy robots</u>) to reduce <u>dispensing errors</u> and free up staff time for more <u>near-patient clinical activities</u>. This led to many hospital pharmacies in the UK implementing a robotic system to automate some, if not all, of its dispensing and supply workload. Now the widespread availability of <u>pharmacy robots</u> in UK hospitals, interfaced with the department's <u>pharmacy system</u>, opens up the possibility of a seamless, <u>closed loop process</u> for the supply of medicines in hospitals, once EP systems are in place and fully integrated with pharmacy systems.

Development of Medicines Information Services and Their Integration with EP Systems

Hospital <u>medicines information services</u> (formerly referred to in the UK context as drug information services) were established in the UK, following the publication of the <u>Noel Hall Report</u> in 1970, which indicated that hospital pharmacists had an important advisory function concerning the medicines that they supplied [55]. During the 1970s, drug information services were established in the UK at regional and local level, staffed by hospital pharmacists, and often working closely with the hospital library. <u>Medicines Information services</u> provide information about medicines to healthcare professionals and patients. Information may be provided in a proactive way – production of local guidelines and bulletins on new medicines and <u>evidence-based medicine</u>, the prescribing of medicines in a rational manner – or in a reactive way – responding to medicine-related enquires submitted by telephone, e-mail or in writing.

For many years, <u>medicines information pharmacists</u> answered medicines-related enquiries and provided information to hospital <u>drug and therapeutics committees</u>, largely based on evaluation of paper-based reference sources, mainly <u>pharmaceutical industry</u> information, the primary medical literature and national prescribing guidelines, such as the <u>Drug & Therapeutics Bulletin</u> and the <u>Medicines Resource Centre (MeReC) Bulletin</u>. These paper sources were supplemented by dial-up online services, such as the US National Library of Medicine <u>Medline</u> service on DataStar and microfiche based products, such as the UK pharmacy service compiled <u>PharmLine</u> and the <u>Iowa Drug Information Service (IDIS)</u>.

However, during the 1990s, there was a shift towards universal availability of medical information in electronic form. This was brought about by two main factors: (a) the increasing use of the CD-ROM as a publication format by medical publishers, and (b) the development and acceptance of the internet as a repository of medical information. This led to the trend of standard medical reference sources, such as the British National Formulary, being made available on hospital intranet sites, for perusal in electronic format, and the development of specialist <u>medicines information internet sites</u>, such as UKMI/UKMICentral and the National Electronic Library of Medicine (NELM) (formerly druginfozone). As well as being used for current awareness, these sites are used for the sharing of hospital derived or compiled information lists (for example, stability information for fridge medicines left out of the fridge).

Due to the ready availability of medicines information in electronic form, from official and ephemeral sources alike, there is the possibility of comprehensive use of <u>electronic medicines information</u>, from networked local sources or internet sources, in future EP applications, at the clinician workstation at the point of care. This will be discussed in detail in the forthcoming chapter on Data Support.

EP Systems and Oncology Systems

The historical development of oncology and hematology prescribing systems represents a special case within the electronic prescribing initiative. Systems for electronic prescribing and dissemination of prescriptions for oncology and hematology patients have already been developed, as part of departmental systems designed for oncology/hematology clinic management. Generally speaking, these systems have been designed to manage the entire patient pathway through an oncology referral, including diagnosis and disease scoring, patient scheduling (incorporating local regulatory requirements, such as the UK NHS 2-week wait rule), pathology test result monitoring, protocol based prescribing, post-cycle toxicity monitoring, pharmacy preparative functions (worksheets and labels) and documentation management. Such systems are now well developed to meet the needs of current clinical practice and management reporting requirements and, as such, are much further ahead, in terms of available functionality, than EP systems for general medicine.

The reasons for this are as follows:

(a) oncology/hematology treatment clinics represent a discrete, well-defined area of clinical practice, where there is very little overlap with other areas of medicine. Development of these systems has thus been on a "silo" basis, as with other healthcare software initiatives.

(b) prescribing for oncology and hematology is distinct from other forms of prescribing as it is largely based on agreed protocols, to which certain well-defined adjustments can be made. Automated systems are therefore an obvious choice for the management of protocol-based prescribing.

(c) the drugs used in chemotherapy are often highly toxic and doses are critical. This is a major driver in the use of automated systems for risk management, to reduce risks that may be introduced by human calculation errors, or failure to heed monitoring results.

(d) the drugs used in chemotherapy usually require specialist compounding/assembly in the pharmacy department. An automated system helps to ensure that worksheets and labels conform to legal requirements and good manufacturing practice requirements.

A number of systems have been developed to meet oncology clinic management requirements and many of these have electronic prescribing and records management functions for chemotherapy and/or radiotherapy prescribing. The Inhealth Systems/Torex/iSOFT suite of applications for oncology, radiotherapy and palliative care management – OPMAS, RCAS and PCAS respectively – were developed and implemented at various sites in the UK between 1987 and 2004. Newer, comprehensive systems include ChemoCare from Clinisys, and MedOncology, from Varian. In addition, the US system IMPAQ has gained considerable ground in the UK market.

In 2005, the UK Government announced its intention to bring forward the electronic prescribing initiative for oncology and cancer care. The rationale for this was that EP systems for oncology would help to resolve the issues of "post-code" pre-scribing of expensive chemotherapy agents and immunomodulators in oncology, and a perceived lack of information governance in oncology prescribing and cancer health outcomes. Consequently, the UK Connecting for Health program – then the National Programme for IT – released a short to medium term specification for oncology systems [56], much of which has since been developed by the oncology specialist software vendors, such as Clinisys and Varian. In 2006, as a national che-motherapy EP solution was still a long way away in the CfH roadmap, CfH under-took a benchmarking process, in which it evaluated a number of existing oncology management solutions from specialist vendors. The Clinisys Chemocare system was given the highest rating in this benchmarking process.

There is little published research on the use of chemotherapy specialist EP sys-tems. Small et al. [57] studied the rate of prescribing errors in a prospective audit of 1941 chemotherapy prescriptions at the Norfolk & Norwich Hospital, Norwich, UK, comparing paper prescriptions and those generated by a chemotherapy pre-scribing system. They found that EP resulted in a 42% reduction in error rate, and that errors occurred in 12% of computerized prescriptions, compared with 20% of paper prescriptions. Interestingly, they found that there was a significant difference in the rates of errors between three prescribers, regardless of the system used, sug-gesting that prescriber training may be an important factor in error reduction, regard-less of the mode of prescribing.

Traer and Madhavan [58] studied the adoption of EP systems into UK clinical settings, especially into cancer networks, in a survey of cancer network lead pharmacists in the UK. They found that, while only 8% of respondents used gen-eral EP system, 32% used chemotherapy EP systems. The authors found that there was considerable national variance in the types of system available, which is unsurprising given the historical development of chemotherapy system use in the UK, and that more coordination was essential to ensure the development of quality systems.

The Development of Consolidated Electronic Medicines Management Systems in Hospitals

As has been discussed, hospitals have implemented a number of different systems for electronic medicines management on a discrete, departmental basis. Hospitals often seek interfaces between these different systems. Furthermore, one of the goals of regional or national healthcare IT program is to develop holistic solutions, which cover all aspects of a healthcare provider's business processes, and which may be rolled out uniformly across a number of hospitals. A suggested architecture for a consolidated EP system, which would address all aspects of a hospital's medicines management needs, is shown in Fig. 2.2.

The benefits that such an architecture might confer are discussed in Chap. 3.

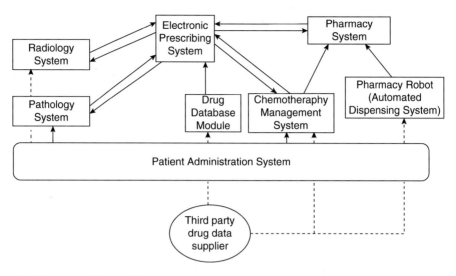

Fig. 2.2 E-prescribing architecture

Barriers to Implementation of EP Systems

There is a consensus on both sides of the Atlantic that the implementation of EP systems is a desirable development, and there are initiatives in both the US and the UK to bring about and incentivize greater adoption of EP systems by healthcare providers. Nevertheless, it is apparent from a review of the historical development of EP systems that various factors play a part in EP system adoption and innovation – and that some of these factors can lead to barriers to system implementation in specific organizations, or in particular healthcare economies.

Some of these are human factors – social and psychological factors – and have been discussed in the previous chapter on the philosophical issues surrounding electronic prescribing. However, some of these are regulatory, financial and political factors, and will be considered here. A number of studies have examined the potential barriers to adoption of healthcare IT applications in general [59, 60] and these factors are equally applicable to EP systems. These factors would include:

(a) High <u>financial costs</u> of installation of EP systems. As well as the actual installation of the EP software and the technology platform (servers, network, desktop computers, palm PCs and PDAs), consideration needs to be given to time spent on site by IT vendor personnel for <u>project management</u>, <u>configuration</u> and <u>testing</u> purposes. If there is not a clear business model for <u>benefits realization</u>, it may be hard for provider organizations to justify the high costs of an EP implementation.

(b) Lack of <u>intraoperability</u> with other systems. Intraoperability – the ability of an EP system to communicate effectively with other IT systems within a healthcare provider organization – is an important deliverable for IT systems, and lack of interoperability, either due to a lack of communication standards, or due to software inadequacies, is a major disincentive for investment in such systems, especially in those countries where regional or national healthcare IT program are pending.

(c) Security and Privacy Issues. Concerns of healthcare professionals and patients about the security of healthcare IT systems have been well-documented both in the professional literature and the popular press. Security has been a controversial issue during the course of the English Connecting for Health healthcare IT program, although some have commented that clinicians' concerns over confidentiality have simply been a means of resisting any interference with their professional interests [61]. Nevertheless, implementers need to consider carefully the local security of their systems, especially if wireless networks are in use. Security is, in fact, a potential benefit of EP systems, and will be discussed as such in the next chapter.

(d) Legal Issues. A wide variety of legal issues can influence the adoption of EP systems. These include:

- the laws governing the prescription and supply of medicines. For example, for many years, the development of EP systems in the UK was impeded by the fact that UK law required a prescription to be signed by hand.
- the laws concerning intellectual property and licensing. For example, there may be a problem with the operation of an EP system, if licenses and permissions to use subsidiary software applications are not in place.
- the laws concerning medical negligence. Fear of negligence proceedings in a highly litigious society may prove a disincentive to implementers of EP systems.
- the laws concerning antitrust. In the US, until recently, the anti-kickback legislation has prevented third parties, such as healthcare providers and insurance payers, from investing in EP software for associated physicians, thus slowing the adoption of EP systems.

Many of these legal issues can be offset by initiatives by governments and government agencies to reform the relevant legislation or to provide new legal provisions, with the specific purpose of encouraging EP implementation, in the public interest.

(e) Failure of software vendors to produce acceptable systems, within agreed timescales. It is widely recognized that not all organizations in the healthcare IT market place are able to provide or install software that is fit for purpose for every application. This is especially the case with electronic prescribing, which is arguably one of the more innovative and complex areas of healthcare IT. There may be a number of reasons for this. Firstly, it is widely understood that the awarding of large contracts to healthcare IT vendors is based more on marketing and commercial factors, rather than on proven expertise and delivery track-record for all the deliverables under negotiation. Secondly, IT vendors may not have the relevant domain expertise available in-house, or may not have the political will to recruit and retain such expertise. Thirdly, many international software suppliers will attempt to adapt software developed in one country, for use in another country. A typical scenario is that software designed for the US market is poorly adapted for use in the UK. This may lead to a composite system, whose design is not adequate for either context, when the better course of action would have been to undertake a lengthier, substantive redesign process, to produce a core product that can be appropriately configured to each healthcare market. Fourthly, many IT companies offshore their design and development facilities, which may hamper the software production process, especially if there is substantial iterations in the testing process, or scope-creep in the software requirements.

Conclusion

To date, there has been a track record of innovation and research with EP systems in the US, the UK, mainland Europe and Australia. In the UK and the US, such innovation has been stimulated by an increasing understanding of the benefits of EP systems. While EP system innovation in the UK has been slow, a number of UK hospitals have developed e-discharge applications, to automate the discharge process, and to deliver benefits in this area. Often, the ease with which EP systems are accepted within local healthcare provider organizations depends on factors that are specific to those organizations, such as how the systems can be linked into other pharmacy IT systems. Some areas of functionality – most notably, chemotherapy clinic management – are further advanced than EP in general. Furthermore, a number of factors have been identified as potential barriers to adoption of EP systems.

References

1. Kohn LT, Corrigan JM, Donaldson MD, editors. To err is human: building a safer health system. Washington, DC: National Academy Press; 1999.
2. Institute of Medicine. Crossing the quality chasm: a new health system for the 21st century. Washington, DC: National Academy Press; 2001.
3. Mosley-Williams A, Williams C. Computer applications in clinical practice. Curr Opin Rheumatol. 2005;17:124–8.
4. Shapiro JP. Industry preaches safety in Pittsburgh. US News & World Report. 2000:56.
5. Bates DW, Gawande AA. Improving safety with information technology. N Engl J Med. 2003;348:2526–34.
6. Bell DS, Friedman MA. E-prescribing and the medicare modernization act of 2003. Health Aff. 2005;24:1159–69.
7. Johnston ME, Langton KB, et al. Effects of computer-based clinical decision support systems on clinician performance and patient outcome: a critical appraisal of research. Ann Intern Med. 1994;120:135–42.
8. Hunt DL, Haynes RB, et al. Effects of computer-based clinical decision support systems on physician performance and patient outcomes. J Am Med Assoc. 1998;280:1339–46.
9. Teich JM, Hurley JF, Beckley RF, Aranow M. Design of an easy-to-use physician order entry system with support for nursing and ancillary departments. Proc Annu Symp Comput Appl Med Care. 1992;16:99–103.
10. Bates DW, Leape L, et al. Effect of computerized physician order entry and a team intervention on prevention of serious medication errors. J Am Med Assoc. 1998;280:1311–6.
11. Bates DW, Teich JM, et al. The impact of computerized physician order entry on medication error prevention. J Am Med Informatics Assoc. 1999;6:313–21.

12. Tierney WM, Miller ME, et al. Physician inpatient order writing on microcomputer workstations: effects on resource utilisation. J Am Med Assoc. 1993;269:379–83.
13. Spencer DC, Leininger A, et al. Effect of a computerized prescriber order entry system on reported medication errors. Am J Health Syst Pharm. 2005;62:416–9.
14. Mekhjian HS, Kumar RR, et al. Immediate benefits realized following implementation of physician order entry at an academic medical center. J Am Med Informatics Assoc. 2002;9:529–39.
15. Koppel R, Metlay JD, et al. Role of computerized physician order entry systems in facilitating medication errors. J Am Med Assoc. 2005;293:1197–203.
16. Stone W, Smith B, et al. Impact of a computerized physician order entry system. J Am Coll Surg. 2009;208(5):960–7.
17. Devine E, Williams E, et al. Prescriber and staff perceptions of an electronic prescribing system in primary care: a qualitative assessment. BMC Med Inform Decis Mak. 2010;10:72.
18. Moniz T, Seger A, et al. Addition of electronic prescription transmission to computerized prescriber order entry: effect on dispensing errors in community pharmacies. Am J Health Syst Pharm. 2011;68:158–63.
19. Anon. E-Prescribing would help hospitals control infection. Pharm J. 2007;278:389.
20. Summers V, Association of Scottish Chief Pharmacists. Electronic prescribing – the way forward. Pharm J. 2000;265:834.
21. Sanghani P. Hospitals must embrace electronic prescribing. Pharm J. 2011;286:331.
22. Goundrey-Smith SJ. Is electronic prescribing a holy grail? Pharm J. 2004;272:412.
23. Moule G. Electronic prescribing – will it ever happen? Guild Healthc Pharma J. 2002:20.
24. Gross Z. What it means to staff when hospitals are ahead in electronic prescribing. Pharm J. 2002;268:679.
25. Curtis C, Ford NG. Paperless electronic prescribing in a district general hospital. Pharm J. 1997;259:734–5.
26. Fowlie F, Bennie M, et al. Evaluation of an electronic prescribing and administration system in a British hospital. Pharm J. 2000;265(Suppl):R16.
27. Gray S, Smith J. Practice report – electronic prescribing in Bristol. Healthc Pharm. 2004:20–2.
28. Clark C. Information technology in action. Hosp Pharm. 2002;9:109–12.
29. Foot R, Taylor L. Electronic prescribing and patient records – getting the balance right. Pharm J. 2005;274:210–2.
30. Beard R, Candlish C. Is electronic prescribing the best system for preventing pharmacy errors? Br J Healthc Comput Info Manage. 2007;24:15–8.
31. Franklin BD, O'Grady K, et al. The impact of a closed-loop electronic prescribing and administration system on prescribing errors, administration errors and staff time: a before and after study. Qual Saf Health Care. 2007;16:279–84.
32. Nightingale PG, Adu D, et al. Implementation of rules-based computerised bedside prescribing and administration: intervention study. Br Med J. 2000;320:750–3.
33. Slee A. E-prescribing in Birmingham. Presented at the Guild of Healthcare Pharmacists/ United Kingdom Clinical Pharmacy Association Information Technology Interest Group (ITIG) seminar. Birmingham, UK. 2010. http://www.ghp.org.uk/ContentFiles/ghpitig10a.pps
34. Fidler B, Anderson C. Implementing EPMA: Experience at King's College Hospital. Presented at the Guild of Healthcare Pharmacists/United Kingdom Clinical Pharmacy Association Information Technology Interest Group (ITIG) seminar. Birmingham, UK. 2009. http://www.ghp.org.uk/ContentFiles/ghpitig0911f.pps. Accessed in December 2011.
35. Heed A. Newcastle Hospitals Electronic Evolution. Presented at the Guild of Healthcare Pharmacists/ United Kingdom Clinical Pharmacy Association Information Technology Interest Group (ITIG) seminar. Birmingham, UK. 2010. http://www.ghp.org.uk/ContentFiles/ghpitig10b.pps. Accessed in December 2011.
36. Cornford T, Savage I, et al. Learning lessons from electronic prescribing implementations in secondary care. Stud Health Technol Inform. 2010;160:233–7.
37. Makinen M, Forsstrom J, et al. A European survey on the possibilities and obstacles of electronic prescriptions in cross-border healthcare. Telemed J E-Health. 2006;12:484–9.
38. Rubio Fernandez M, Aldaz Frances R, et al. Computer-aided electronic prescribing in Spanish hospitals (abstract only). Farm Hosp. 2005;29:236–40.

39. Llopis Salvia P, Sanchez Alcaraz A, et al. Integral computerisation of healthcare for inpatients. Impact on primary care activities (abstract only). Farm Hosp. 2003;27:231–9.
40. Nielsen EW, Dybwik K. Drug interactions in an intensive care unit (abstract only). Tidsskr Nor Laegeforen. 2004;124:2907–8.
41. Bonnabry P, Despont-Gros C, et al. A risk analysis method to evaluate the impact of a computerized provider order entry system on patient safety. J Am Med Inform Assoc. 2008;15:453–60.
42. Colpaert K, Decruyenaere J. Computerised physician order entry in critical care. Best Pract Res Clin Anaesthesiol. 2009;23:27–38.
43. Niazkhani Z, Pirnejad H, et al. Computerised provider order entry system – does it support the inter-professional medication process? Methods Inf Med. 2010;49:20–7.
44. Van Doormal J, Van den Bemt P, et al. The influence that electronic prescribing has on medication errors and preventable adverse drug events: an interrupted time series study. J Am Med Inform Assoc. 2009;16:816–25.
45. Buising KL, Thursky KA, et al. Electronic antibiotic stewardship – reduced consumption of broad-spectrum antibiotics using a computerised antimicrobial system in a hospital setting. J Antimicrob Chemother. 2008;62:608–16.
46. Sintchenko V, Coiera E, et al. Decision support systems for antibiotic prescribing. Curr Opin Infect Dis. 2008;21:573–9.
47. Baysari MT, Westbrook J, et al. The role of computerised decision support in reducing errors in selecting medicines for prescription: narrative review. Drug Saf. 2011;34:289–98.
48. Magrabi F, Li SY, Day RO, Coiera E. Errors and electronic prescribing; a controlled laboratory study to examine task complexity and interruption effects. J Am Med Inform Assoc. 2010;17:575–83.
49. Clark C. Information technology in action. Hosp Pharm. 2002;9:109–12.
50. Pepperrell M, Patel N. E-Discharge Summary. Presented at the Guild of Healthcare Pharmacists/ United Kingdom Clinical Pharmacy Association Information Technology Interest Group (ITIG) seminar. Birmingham, UK. 2010. http://www.ghp.org.uk/ContentFiles/ghpitig10e.pps. Accessed in December 2011.
51. Lewis R. What's wrong with a piece of paper? The Electronic Transfer of Care. Presented at the guild of Healthcare Pharmacists/United Kingdom Clinical Pharmacy Association Information Technology Interest Group (ITIG) seminar. Birmingham, UK. 2009. http://www.ghp.org.uk/ ContentFiles/ghpitig0911e.pps. Accessed in December 2011.
52. Kirby J, Barker B, et al. A prospective case control study of the benefits of electronic discharge summaries. J Telemed Telecare. 2006;12(S1):20–1.
53. Rose D. E-Discharge with Formulary Control. Presented at the Guild of Healthcare Pharmacists/ United Kingdom Clinical Pharmacy Association Information Technology Interest Group (ITIG) seminar. Birmingham, UK. 2011. http://www.ghp.org.uk/ContentFiles/ghpitig11e.pps. Accessed in December 2011.
54. Audit Commission. A spoonful of sugar – medicines management in NHS hospitals. London: Audit Commission; 2001.
55. Smith SJ, Bottle R. Use of information sources by drug information pharmacists. Pharm J. 1994;253:499–501.
56. NHS Connecting for Health. Cancer services electronic prescribing system – output based specification for immediate/medium term use. 2005. NPfIT-EP-BS-0006.01. Accessed in December 2011.
57. Small M, Barrett A, et al. The impact of computerised prescribing on error rate in a department of oncology/haematology. J Oncol Pharm Pract. 2008;14:181–7.
58. Traer E, Madhavan K. Electronic prescribing and transfer/discharge summaries: a survey of UK cancer networks. Pharm J. 2010;284:453–4.
59. Anderson JG. Social, ethical and legal barriers to E-health. Int J Med Informatics. 2007;76:480–3.
60. Smith AD. Barriers to accepting e-prescribing in the USA. Int J Health Care Qual Assur Inc Leadersh Health Serv. 2006;19:158–80.
61. Barker S. The poisoned chalice. Pharm Mag. 2007:33–4, 36.

Chapter 3
Organization Benefits of Electronic Prescribing

The potential for IT systems and applications to facilitate <u>changes in working practices</u> by automating mundane, logical processes is now well-recognized throughout the business world. Indeed, much commercial <u>system design</u> methodology now seeks to model data and <u>business processes</u>, using tools such as UML diagrams, in order to design software that is the "solution" to the business challenge, regardless of past practices and procedures. Thus the introduction of a new software solution can lead to an organization meeting its business objectives more efficiently, with a paradigm shift – a radical change in working practices – for those who are involved in the business area.

Healthcare IT applications such as electronic patient records, EP and order communications have led to a paradigm shift in working practices, and indeed professional role, for many healthcare professionals. For pharmacists, this has been described as a move away from product and process-centered work, towards patient-centered work [1], and will be discussed in greater detail in a later chapter.

Principles of Business Process Redesign

Analysis of business processes is essentially part of the design phase of software production, and is therefore properly within the remit of <u>software vendors</u>. Nevertheless, implementers should be aware of the general principles of business analysis, <u>business process modeling</u> and <u>business process redesign</u> for a number of reasons:

(a) In practice, many healthcare software providers do not have adequate clinical <u>domain expertise</u> in-house, and will seek input from clinical professionals within the NHS when implementing a system at a particular site, via <u>user groups</u> and, in some cases, at the software design phase.

(b) Many modern Windows-based systems have a vast range of <u>configuration options</u> embedded within them. Furthermore, the more complex the processes

S. Goundrey-Smith, *Principles of Electronic Prescribing*, Health Informatics,   47
DOI 10.1007/978-1-4471-4045-0_3, © Springer-Verlag London 2012

being supported, the greater the need for different configuration and installation options. For a system designed for commercial distribution, <u>configuration options</u> are useful as they increase the number of customer sites that a system where a system can be installed without major code changes and enhancements. <u>Configuration</u> of software is desirable from the implementer's perspective, whereas <u>customization</u> of software (where a particular build of software is provided for one customer) is not [2]. This is for three reasons: (i) customization of software is costly to the customer, (ii) customized software may not be adequately supported by a vendor, and (iii) further changes would be controlled by the vendor, not the customer.

(c) An appreciation of the <u>business processes</u> being modeled, and the assumptions taken when designing the software to support those processes, provide implementers with a valuable insight into why the software was designed as it was.

Consequently, there are a number of important principles of <u>business process redesign</u> that need to be considered by implementers of EP systems and associated healthcare software applications.

Firstly, within an enterprise or organizational unit, as many of the <u>business processes</u> as possible should be modeled in order to provide a solution that is holistic, and that covers the vast majority of business scenarios that might arise in the organization. A single system covering a range of business processes will be more efficient and consistent in its operation because common server platforms, data platforms and application algorithms will be in use.

Given the range of different types of business scenario and use case that can occur across healthcare, it is difficult in practice to produce systems that are truly universal in their scope. It is primarily for this reason, as well as for reasons of system ownership, that traditionally in healthcare, systems have developed in a "silo" manner as individual departments and professional groups have sought to automate their processes in a "bottom up" approach. Consequently, many healthcare software vendors have taken a modular approach, where a PAS can be supplemented with an order communications module, an electronic prescribing module etc – such as the Meditech system. Furthermore, in any particular healthcare enterprise, there may be reasons why a system may not cover all business areas – for example, where a satellite hospital or remote unit does not have full connectivity or system availability for communications or <u>infrastructure</u> reasons.

<u>Regional or national healthcare IT projects</u>, where they are successful, provide opportunities for large, highly configurable systems to be deployed, which aim to address as many healthcare business processes as possible. Indeed, many <u>software vendors</u> are seeking to provide products based on "<u>service oriented architecture</u>" where the structure of the system is based on the services it is intended to support, and processes that are common to all functions (e.g. <u>terminology</u> and <u>decision support</u>) are provided by single engines, which are integrated with the various service units within the system. While <u>service oriented architecture</u> is of great benefit in supporting a large range of use cases in an efficient and consistent manner, it confers uniformity on the system that may render it easier to interchange

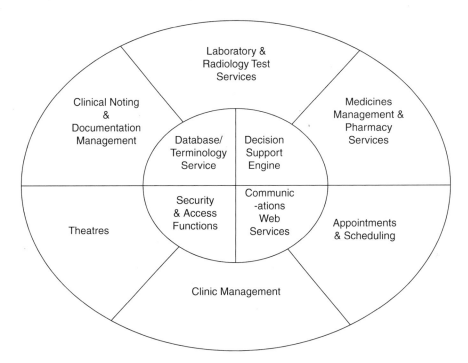

Fig. 3.1 Service oriented architecture (SOA). A notional hospital information system based on SOA. The specialist functional modules in the *outer circle* are serviced by the core components

with another similar architecture, which has major commercial implications for software vendors (Fig. 3.1).

Secondly, the scope of the business processes being supported must be clearly defined. Given the vast number of business processes and scenarios that are in operation in a healthcare setting, it is inevitable that some processes will not be able to be supported by a single system. This may be for infrastructure reasons, or because an alternative system, or a legacy system, is already in place, which the organization does not wish to replace, or which is not easily replicated. In this situation, it is important to define the scope of the new system clearly. It is also important to have a clear understanding of the type and capability of any interfaces that will be required with existing systems. This is important, given the way that, historically, systems in healthcare have developed in a "silo" manner (silo development). Furthermore, interface requirements are of particular significance in medicines management since, in order to provide full business process management, an EP system would need to interface with a PAS, a pharmacy system, and an automated dispensing system (pharmacy robot) via the pharmacy system. Issues surrounding interfaces of this type will be discussed in detail later in the chapter.

Thirdly, the significance of business processes must be clearly understood in their context before a software solution can be designed to support them. Take, for example, the UK practice of 28-day dispensing, or "one stop" dispensing. It is important that an EP system has the functions to support 28 day dispensing (a 28 day supply flag for items, with a reorder after 21 days algorithm etc), but it is essential to realize that the rationale for 28-day dispensing is to prevent duplicate dispensing and thus streamline the discharge process. This awareness ensures that all associated functionality – e.g. discharge functions – will be designed and linked in appropriately.

Fourthly, and most significantly, it is essential when implementing a new system that business processes are not reverse engineered to match the system design, or technological capability available, rather than the software designed and configured to support current – and, most importantly, emerging – business processes. On the one hand, the appropriate technology must be available to ensure that an application can be deployed across an enterprise without any loss of performance; some early EP programs in the US failed because the technology used was not scaleable [3]. On the other hand, technology may fail to deliver benefits if it does not meet needs, or it requires that practice is altered to accommodate system use [1]. Indeed, experience from the US suggests that healthcare providers need a technology strategy to ensure that technology supports the organization's goals, rather than fitting business processes around the available technology [4]. The avoidance of reverse-engineering is particularly important for EP systems, given the observation that EP systems are "sociotechnical innovations" [5] where the computer and human components contribute to the overall performance of the system.

Appropriate use of electronic systems to support current and emerging business processes will be facilitated by highly configurable systems, use of service oriented architecture and the involvement of clinical professionals and domain experts in their design.

Medicines Management in Hospitals: Existing Business Processes

However, prior to any discussion of the appropriate design of EP systems and their impact on hospital business processes, it would be beneficial to describe the way the prescribing and medicines supply process has taken place in hospitals to date.

Traditionally, in a hospital, medicines for inpatients have been prescribed on a medicine administration chart, commonly referred to as a drug chart, and sometimes called a "Kardex".

An example of the layout of a drug chart is shown in Fig. 3.2.

The drug chart will have sections of the page allocated to prescriptions of:

- Regular medicines. These are medicines that are given on a regular basis, at set administration times. An example of this would be: Amoxicillin 500 mg Capsules – one to be taken three times a day at 08.00, 14.00 and 22.00.
- When required (PRN) medicines. These are medicines that are given only when required to treat acute symptoms, and are generally medicines such as analgesics,

ONCE ONLY DRUGS AND PREMEDICATION DRUGS

Approved Drug Name	Dose	Route	Prescriber Signature	Time to be Given	Date to be Given	Date and Time Given	Given by: Check by:	Pharmacy Supply

REGULAR PRESCRIPTIONS Date:

			Regular Times / Other Times															
Approved Drug Name	Dose		0600															
			1000															
Signature	Date	Frequency:	1200															
			1400															
Special Directions	Pharmacy Supply:	Pharmacy Supply: / Pharmacist Check:	1800															
			2200															

VARIABLE TIMES/DOSES

Approved Drug Name	Dose	Route	Date												
Signature	Date	Pharmacy Supply	Time												
			Dose												
Special Directions	Pharmacist Check	Pharmacy Supply	Initial												
			Check												

RECORD OF ONCE ONLY STANDING ORDER DRUGS/FLUID GIVEN

Approved Drug Name	Dose	Route	Signature of Nurse/Midwife	Date	Time	Given by:	Check by:	Pharm Supply

CONTINUOUS INTRAVENOUS/ SUBCUTANEOUS DRUG INFUSION THERAPHY

Approved Drug Name	Diluent	Volume	Route	Date												
				Time												
Concentration (mg/ml etc.)	Flow Rate (ml/hr)		Supply	Rate												
Prescribers Signature	Date		Supply	Initial/ Check												
Special Directions	Pump Code:		Pharmacist Check	Volume Infused												

Fig. 3.2 Medicine administration charts

antiemetics and laxatives. They are not given at set administration times, but the time and date of each dose is recorded on the chart when it is given. An example of a PRN medicine would be: acetaminophen/paracetamol 500 mg tablets – one or two to be taken every 4–6 h as required for pain.

- Once only (Statim) medicines. These are medicines that are given as a single dose, with no instruction to repeat the dose. These medicines may be routinely given, for example, vaccines, or may be given in relation to a particular procedure that has been, or is about to be, performed. An example of a once only medicine would be: Diazepam 10 mg by intravenous injection (as a premedication before an operation).

- Fluids. These are large volume infusions routinely given in hospital for the purpose of hydration or plasma replacement, in clinical situations where they are needed. A fluid is essentially a once only order, but it is given over a period of time, and the flow rate of the fluid is set using a burette on the intravenous giving set. An example would be: Sodium Chloride Infusion 0.9% 1 l, to be given over 6 h.

- Continuous Infusions. These are intravenous infusions that are given at a fixed or variable rate to treat a specific disease. Unlike fluids, continuous infusions will be small volume (250 ml or less) and will consist of medicines with specific pharmacological activity. Furthermore, because of the potent effects of the drugs used, they are usually delivered by a syringe driver, which will maintain a more accurate flow rate than can be achieved with the burette on a fluid giving set. An example of a continuous infusion would be: Isosorbide Dinitrate 50 mg in 50 ml Infusion, given at a variable rate of between 2 and 4 mg/h for the treatment of ischemic (angina) pain.

When prescribing a medicine, the prescriber writes the details on the drug chart, and the various boxes on each section in the drug chart prompts the prescriber to include all relevant details for a particular order type. The prescription is then signed by the prescriber.

The drug chart is then used as the basis for medicine supply and medicines administration in the hospital. Medicines are supplied against the formulation details on the drug chart, either from ward stock, if a medicine is used regularly on a ward, or direct from the pharmacy. Pharmacists make prescription-related enquiries based on the details on the drug chart, and make any relevant additions or amendments on the chart (traditionally in green pen, in UK hospitals). Nursing staff then administer the medicine to the patient according to the detail on the drug chart. Each administration of a medicine is recorded by the nurse administering the medicine – the date, time and initials of the administering nurse are recorded. If a regular, or scheduled, prescription is not administered, an agreed missed dose code is placed in the administration box, instead of the nurse's initials. This indicates the reason why a dose is not administered – for example, the patient refused the medicine, the patient is "nil by mouth" or the medicine is not available. For fluids and intravenous medicines, there is the facility to record that an infusion was stopped due to a blockage in the giving set, or extravasation – where the intravenous cannula has come out of the patient's vein, and the drug is leaking into the surrounding tissues.

While a patient is an inpatient, all medication will be recorded on the drug chart, together with a record of administration, with the exception of anesthetics and perioperative medication, and possibly some departmental investigations. However, when the patient is discharged, a discharge prescription is written (this is sometimes referred to as a "to take out/away" (TTO/TTA) prescription) and sent to the pharmacy to be prepared. The discharge prescription is usually completed on a separate form, in duplicate or triplicate, and includes the attending clinician's diagnosis, treatment and planned follow-up/care plan.

The drug chart/Kardex system of recording medicine prescribing and administration has remained unchanged for 40 or 50 years [2]. Nevertheless, in practical terms, there are many problems associated with it.

(a) Because prescriptions are handwritten – often in a hurry by busy clinicians – they may be illegible or incomplete. Alternatively, in patients with large numbers of medicines, there may be inadvertent duplications.
(b) Nursing staff may have to query prescriptions before they administer them, leading to inefficiencies in the medicines administration process.
(c) The drug chart can be lost. If there are two or more charts, they may become separated from each other.
(d) Medicine administration may be delayed when a drug chart is not on the ward for any reason – for example, when a patient is having an investigation in another department, and the chart has gone with them, or the chart is at the pharmacy.
(e) The drug chart cannot easily be reviewed alongside results of tests and other monitoring investigations.
(f) The drug chart cannot be viewed remotely by a clinician or other health professional; the clinician has to attend the ward or department to view the patient chart.
(g) For a medicine that is not ward stock to be ordered from the pharmacy, either the chart must go to the pharmacy department (leading to situation described in d, above) or a pharmacist must transcribe the prescription details onto a pharmacy order list (with the potential for transcription errors)
(h) The discharge prescription generation and fulfillment process represents a major workload for the pharmacy department in many UK hospitals. There are many inefficiencies in the process that lead to delays in patient discharge, difficulties with bed management and low staff morale, as discussed in Chap. 2.

Organizational Benefits of EP

Electronic prescribing systems can offer possible solutions to all of these problems with the current medicine supply process, and therefore can promote efficiency in the medicine prescribing process and medicines administration process in hospital. As mentioned previously, a review of UK EP implementations has identified a number of key benefits with EP systems [6]. They are as follows:

(a) Availability of a fully electronic prescribing history
(b) Improvement in legibility & completeness of prescriptions
(c) Improvement in hospital business processes due to electronic dissemination of prescriptions
(d) Improvement in the quality of prescribing due to the availability of electronic decision support tools at the point of prescribing
(e) A comprehensive audit trail of prescribing decisions made
(f) Reduction in the rate of medication-related errors

All of these benefits impact on the efficiency of the healthcare enterprise, as well as the optimum care and safety of the patient. EP systems have particular organizational benefits in the following areas:

1. <u>Workflow management</u> for <u>clinical users</u> of EP systems
2. Facilitation of a Seamless Pharmaceutical Supply Chain
3. Reduced use of <u>paper and consumables</u>
4. Clinical System <u>Intraoperability</u>
5. Improvement in hospital <u>business processes</u> due to <u>electronic dissemination of prescriptions</u>
6. Contribution of Workflow Improvement to <u>Professional Practice Development</u>
7. <u>Security</u> of prescriptions and prescribing information
8. <u>Quality of care</u> benefits

These issues will be discussed in detail from an organizational and ergonomic perspective.

Workflow Management for Clinical Users of EP Systems

Clinical professionals of all disciplines face a two-fold task in their daily practice in a healthcare environment. On the one hand, they have a <u>duty of care</u> towards their patients, and an obligation to ensure that patients are treated in a way that fulfils <u>legal requirements</u> and <u>ethical requirements</u>, and most closely represents accepted <u>best practice</u> for their profession. On the other hand, there are operational pressures from the healthcare organization to treat patients as quickly and efficiently as possible and to achieve statistical benchmarks and <u>service level targets</u>. Furthermore, these two objectives can sometimes seem to be in opposition; best care of the patient by the practitioner may be at the expense of meeting organizational targets. However, there is a greater chance of both objectives being achieved if workflow for the practitioner – both the prescriber of a medicine and the person administering the medicine – is streamlined by the appropriate use of electronic systems.

For many healthcare systems, designed for use in a busy working environment, the design of the <u>user interface</u> is important. For an application such as electronic prescribing, where there is a need to present complex prescribing information in a way that enables appropriate professional decision making, and to input comprehensive medicine order information in a straightforward and timely manner, <u>user interface design</u> is critical.

Prescribing Workflow Design

The obvious benefit of EP system is a <u>legible and complete prescription</u>, facilitated by the electronic display of that information. Thus, an EP system can ensure that, for every prescription, the following details will be included:

- Medicine
- Form/Formulation
- Strength
- Dose
- Route
- Frequency
- Duration (if applicable)
- Any specific prescribing or administration instructions

The legibility and completeness of prescriptions is beneficial to the working practices of all system users involved in the prescribing, dispensing and administration of medicines. Two UK implementations of EP systems have commented on the positive impact of EP on the legibility and completeness of the prescribing record [7, 8]. In an analysis of 2,180 prescriptions from the Wirral Trust, UK, for legibility and completeness, with reference to hospital standards for prescription writing, based on the British National Formulary, it was found that electronic prescribing significantly improved the legibility and completeness of prescriptions compared with prescribing by hand (p<0.0001). Furthermore, in a recent analysis of the use of an EP system in an ophthalmology day unit, electronic prescriptions resulted in 100% capture of prescription information [9].

In a review of EP experience at Wirral, presented at the British Pharmaceutical Conference in 1999 [10], Farrar indicated that the use of EP at the Wirral Hospitals had increased the number of complete and correct doses on medication charts from 17.7% to approaching 100%. However, the record of dose administration was not always complete; often once only prescriptions were completely and correctly prescribed, but no record was made of when they were administered.

The legibility and completeness of an electronic prescription are dependent on other factors. Firstly, the legibility of prescription information on an electronic system in the clinical environment cannot be assumed; it will depend on (a) the design of the screens and forms used to display the data, (b) fonts and styles of text used, (c) graphics and colors used on the screens. The adoption of chart designs and form templates that were already in use in the hospital, as happened in Burton on Trent, UK [11], will facilitate staff familiarization with the system and, as well as having a positive effect on the reduction of prescribing errors and medicine administration errors, will increase staff confidence in the system and the efficiency with which the EP system is used.

Secondly, the completeness of the displayed prescribing history will depend on the completeness of the prescription data captured in the first place. To facilitate adequate prescribing data capture, the database structure should have sufficient granularity, and the medicines data should be sufficiently comprehensive to handle a wide range of complex prescribing scenarios. This is because, in general terms, many prescriptions generated in secondary care are more complex and varied than those in primary care.

For example, a secondary care EP system would need to include:

(a) a comprehensive range of <u>routes</u> (including routes to support <u>enteral feeding</u>)
(b) a comprehensive range of <u>formulation</u> types,
(c) reducing/increasing <u>dose regimens</u> (e.g. prednisolone reducing dose),
(d) <u>loading doses</u> and associated <u>maintenance</u> doses of the same drug (e.g. gentamicin),
(e) alternate <u>routes</u> of administration for the same drug dose (e.g. metoclopramide 10 mg po/pr/im),
(f) <u>complex administration instructions</u> (e.g. co-trimoxazole 960 mg on Monday, Wednesday and Friday). The provision of adequate functionality to allow capture of complex drug orders is important because, in two reports [10, 12], it was found that errors of omission increased after EP implementation, because prescribers found themselves unable to enter certain types of prescription due to the design of the system and the configuration of the drug data.

Other issues associated with data capture concern the use of screen prompts and the use of free text fields. Firstly, it has been demonstrated that functions to prompt the user to fill in each line of the form in the prescribing workflow help to minimize missing information and maximize patient safety [9]. Secondly, in an analysis of 2,914 electronic prescriptions with free text fields, it was found that there were internal data discrepancies in 16.1% of prescriptions, leading to adverse events in 83.8% of cases and severe adverse events in 16.8% of cases [13]. Many of the discrepancies were between structured and free text fields, and the study authors indicated that designers should use free text fields with care in the prescribing workflow.

In addition to the clear display of a <u>prescribing history</u> for a patient, another important issue in facilitating an efficient workflow for the user is the ease of operation of the system. For any EP system, there is a balance between the completeness of data capture during the prescribing process, and ease and <u>usability</u> of the system for the prescriber. A system might have a 12 stage prescribing process to enable the clinician to prescribe a complex regimen, but this may not be acceptable a busy clinician using the system. One way of addressing this issue might be to use <u>pre-defined orders (PDOs)</u> for commonly used prescriptions (e.g. Furosemide 40 mg Tablets – one to be taken each morning), so that the clinician can select a complete medication order in a single process. This approach was used in the pilot at Southmead Hospital, Bristol, UK [7] to speed up the prescribing process and to incorporate implicit <u>decision support</u>, in the form of prescribing guidance. However, use of PDOs may lead to different kinds of error due to incorrect selection of a PDO, or errors within a PDO being propagated inadvertently through large numbers of patient records.

As well as the number of operations required to generate an electronic medicine order, in terms of defining the order details – medicine, form, strength, dose, route, frequency etc – consideration needs to be given to the number of <u>confirmation boxes</u> ("double dares") and warning messages that appear during the workflow for different types of prescribing. It is well recognized that, if a system presents an excessive number of clinical warnings in any particular workflow, especially warnings that are irrelevant to the specific prescribing scenario, the user will begin to ignore the warnings (so-called "<u>warning fatigue</u>").

The need for confirmation boxes may be reduced by the appropriate use of control default options and highlighting, but the risk management implications of these developments need to be considered carefully. Furthermore, due to the increasing granularity of data – both coded data from patient records, and drug data within decision support systems – decision support data providers are now looking at aggregated querying techniques to produce single warning messages that are more intuitive to the particular prescribing scenario. The issues surrounding warning fatigue will be examined in more detail in the decision support section in Chap. 5.

Medicines Administration Workflow

Just as the prescribing workflow of an EP system can affect the efficiency with which clinicians prescribe medicine, so the medicine administration workflow of an EP system can streamline the process of medicines administration in a hospital environment. As with the prescribing workflow, the medicine administration workflow is highly dependent on the user interface and the screen layout.

Some systems have been designed to capture the prescribing history electronically but, rather than providing a real-time on-screen medicines administration system, they have instead produced computer-generated charts based on the electronic prescribing record. There is then the facility to reprint, or overprint, these computer-generated charts, following on from changes to the electronic prescribing history. While such a system avoids the complexities of an electronic medicine administration function, it is fundamentally flawed because the administration system is not part of the system, in real time.

A paper-output EP system has the following problems:

(a) For acute medical wards, where there will be a high turnover of patients, and a high turnover of prescribed medication per patient, it will be impossible to maintain a current set of computer-generated charts for each patient.
(b) It is difficult to define a series of trigger events for chart reprinting that fit all situations
(c) A number of problems with paper charts – e.g. loss or damage to the chart – still apply

For these reasons, it is now well recognized that an EP system must include electronic medicine administration functionality (electronic drug administration, or electronic nurse administration) to provide a satisfactory medicines management system. In order to present the complexities of all prescription types in a concise manner, some EP systems have chosen to design a medicines administration screen that, to a greater or lesser extent, mimics the traditional drug chart or Kardex, with sections for each of the prescription types – regular, when required, once only, fluid and continuous infusions. Figure 3.3 shows the design of a medicines administration screen for scheduled (regular) medicines on an EP system. This allows administration of the medicine within a defined timeframe, and also provides other

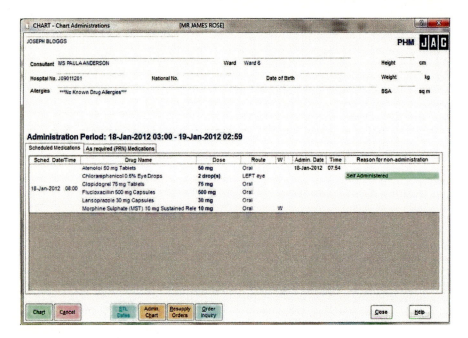

Fig. 3.3 Layout of an EP system medicines administration screen (By kind permission of JAC Computer Services Ltd)

functions to support medicines administration (witnessing for CDs, referential data on the medicine etc.).

In an EP system, the design of the administration screen will facilitate and manage the medicines administration process. For example, the different order types might be displayed on different tabs on screen, so that the nurse can view all active orders according to order type. Scheduled orders – due at a particular time – could be displayed distinctively – for example, highlighted in red. The order could then revert to the standard background once the administration had been recorded (or alternatively show in, for example, green for a set period of time after the administration had been recorded, to indicate that it was a current administration that had recently been done). For regular medicines, there would be a facility to input a user code for the person administering the medicine; for other order types, there should be a facility to record a user code, a date and time of administration and a dose, where a variable dose is required. With all scheduled order types, there should be the facility to record a missed-dose code.

Alternatively, all of the orders scheduled to be given at any given time could be displayed on one administration screen, regardless of order type. The disadvantage of this, however, is that they may not be immediately viewable alongside the whole record of prescribed medication.

Electronic medicine administration has the advantage that it can force users to conform to a general process for medicines administration. However, the underlying rules used by an EP system for electronic medicine administration are potentially complex and would need to be carefully considered, in relation to the established policies and professional practices within a hospital or healthcare provider organization.

Among others, the following issues would need to be considered:

(a) What would be an appropriate time window for highlighting a scheduled prescription as due for administration? For example, with a regular medicine, the system might highlight it in red for an hour either side of the scheduled administration time

(b) What would be an appropriate time window for allowing a scheduled prescription to be administered? For example, with a regular medicine, the system might enable recording of an administration (cells active and highlighted) for an hour either side of the scheduled administration time.

(c) Should once only medicines and fluids display as being administrable as soon as they are electronically signed by the prescriber? If they are not administered, how long should they persist on the administration profile?

(d) Should "lock out" functions exist for when required medicines? For example, the system might disable the prescribing of paracetamol based analgesics more frequently than every 4 h and at doses of more than eight tablets in 24 h.

Other issues that would need to be considered in detail would be the design of administration functions for continuous infusions and controlled drugs, the configuration of missed dose codes and the provision of an on-hold and off-hold facility for items that have been prescribed, but which need to be withheld pending other events, for example pathology test results. The latter function is useful in a number of situations involving elective treatments – for example chemotherapy.

Facilitation of a Seamless Pharmaceutical Supply Chain

Many of the inefficiencies of existing manual prescribing and medicine supply processes in hospitals surround the way in which prescriptions written on the wards are filled with actual medicines from the hospital pharmacy department. Consequently, a direct link between each ward and the pharmacy department, either as different workstations in a networked EP system, or as an interface between an EP hub and a pharmacy system, represents the means for automating order transfer between wards and the pharmacy, and a valuable tool for reducing inefficiency in the pharmacy requisition process. This is shown in the architecture diagram in Chap. 2 (Fig. 2.2).

A conspicuous benefit from a UK perspective is the potential for EP to streamline the discharge process [7]. However, while systems offer a seamless transmission from the ward to the pharmacy, or real-time display of prescribing information in the pharmacy, the total business processes of handing pharmacy supply of discharge prescriptions (TTOs) should be considered. Implementers will need to assess how an EP system can be configured to their established procedures and, alternatively, how their procedures may need to be modified following the introduction of an EP system. An EP system should be able to provide a comprehensive supporting information for each discharge prescription to enable a clinical pharmacist to undertake an initial clinical evaluation (diagnosis, tests performed, care plan etc). It should also provide distinct functions for clinically checking a TTO as a whole, as opposed to individual items on the inpatient prescribing record. Consideration should also be given to how the system might facilitate workflow management within the pharmacy. It is important that all of these factors are considered because they will all contribute to any benefits in terms of staff time efficiency and streamlining of the discharge process. As discussed in Chap. 2, many UK hospitals have already put systems in place to deal with the discharge process ahead of, or instead of, EP systems.

In addition to the way that an EP system can streamline medicine ordering and supply within a hospital, it has been suggested that EP systems can help to facilitate a seamless pharmaceutical supply chain from manufacturer to patient. For over 20 years, hospital pharmacists in many countries have been using departmental pharmacy systems for procurement and stock control of medicines. More recently, automated dispensing systems (pharmacy robots) have been introduced to increase the accuracy of the dispensing process. Furthermore, with the availability of web-based intranets and the associated security technology, together with the growth of e-commerce and the regulatory framework to support it, many pharmaceutical wholesalers are looking to promote e-procurement of medicines by hospitals. Moreover, many hospital pharmacies are seeking to implement e-procurement, with the stock movement and control efficiencies that it can provide.

Consequently, there now exists the means for a seamless pharmaceutical supply chain from the pharmaceutical industry to pharmaceutical wholesalers, and then via central procurement agencies and hospital pharmacies to the patient.

To this end, the baseline specification for the English Connecting for Health electronic prescribing program proposed a number of functionalities that were intended to streamline the medicines supply chain. These included:

(a) an electronic link from the ward to the pharmacy for placing orders
(b) interface with hospital pharmacy systems
(c) automatic escalations for overdue medicines
(d) support for newer stock control methodologies such as 28-day dispensing and patient's own drugs (PODs),
(e) supply chain tracking in real time (viewable by patient), and
(f) medicine costs to be displayed throughout the supply chain.

While many of these requirements may seem straightforward, there are various implications of providing these functions. Firstly, as many implementers have already found out, the interface of an EP system to an (existing) pharmacy system may not be straightforward, in terms of interface building and data configuration. Furthermore, provision of price information for medicines is problematic, both in terms of appropriate adjustments for actual and notional costs, and maintaining the data in real time, throughout the system, at each point of the supply chain. Secondly, supply chain tracking which includes the wholesaler would require involvement of wholesaler systems staff to provide a link between hospital EP systems and NHS e-procurement processes, and the complexities that would involve. Thirdly, provision of supply chain information to patients, as the end-user, would potentially increase the number of disputes between the pharmacy department and wards concerning throughput issues.

It is highly desirable that an EP system should support the various <u>stock control methodologies</u> currently used in hospital pharmacy – <u>28 day dispensing</u>, <u>use of patients' own drugs (PODs)</u> etc. However, as with clinical pharmacy tools, this represents an area that is unique to hospital pharmacy, and pharmacy managers should have an active role in the design of these functions.

Reduced Use of Paper and Consumables

Traditionally, hospital records have been used and stored in a paper format. As well as the clinical notes pages, the records include pro forma results pages for radiology and other departmental investigations and mount sheets for pathology result slips. The records for one patient will have different sections in the <u>clinical notes</u> for each specialty and admission, together with outpatient appointments. As a consequence, the records for a patient who has had a long history of <u>chronic disease</u> and/or <u>multiple acute referrals</u> to clinicians of different specialties may fill several folders and occupy up to 50 cm of shelf-space in A4 format. The difficulties associated with the storage and retrieval of such records have driven the developments in <u>patient administration systems (PAS)</u> and <u>clinical coding</u> over the last 30 years. Specifically, hospital inpatient prescribing records have been recorded on a <u>drug chart</u>, or Kardex, as discussed previously. During any one admission, a patient may have a number of different charts, some of which might be overflow charts with only one or two entries on, prior to the aggregation of the patient's current prescriptions on a single new chart. Multiple drug charts leads to the risk of inadvertent medicine duplication, where a medicine is prescribed in error on more than one chart.

The introduction of electronic prescribing and medicine administration will therefore reduce the amount of consumables used by a health provider – charts, paper, pens etc. Depending on the size of the healthcare provider, the resulting savings may be significant. Nevertheless, while these savings may represent a clear, unambiguous and relatively easily measurable benefit of introducing an EP system, they are insignificant compared to the costs of wasted staff time due to inefficient paper-based systems and processes, and the possible costs of <u>litigation</u> when errors are made, as a result of these inadequate processes. However, unlike savings on <u>paper and consumables</u>, costs for staff time and potential <u>litigation</u> are more difficult to calculate, and it will be tempting for health providers not to attempt to quantify them.

Clinical System Intraoperability

The ability of different clinical systems to interact with each other in an integrated manner is a key factor in the streamlining of healthcare <u>business processes</u> within a hospital or healthcare provider. This is especially the case given the disparate nature of many business processes within a healthcare enterprise, and the <u>silo development</u> of individual departmental systems in the past.

In a number of UK EP implementations, authors have commented on the ability of an EP system to provide a complete and comprehensive <u>prescribing history</u>, which is <u>interfaced</u> with the hospital <u>electronic patient record (EPR)</u> system [7, 11, 14]. This reduces the number of lost or absent medication records, facilitates remote electronic prescribing and enables the easy production of hard copy <u>discharge prescriptions</u> and other supporting information from different locations. A US study has shown that, where an EP system is integrated with an EPR system (in line with the meaningful use requirements), the physician is more likely to consult the patient's prescribing history than when EP is provided as a stand-alone system [15].

With EP system interfaces or integration, there is therefore the potential for transferability of the <u>prescribing history</u> to and from other systems. For example, this enables electronic prescriptions to be routed to the hospital pharmacy departmental system, to streamline the medicine supply process, as discussed previously. This would also enable <u>pathology test</u> orders to be triggered from within the EP system, and sent to the <u>pathology system</u>, and for <u>pathology test results</u> to be posted to the EP system.

As mentioned previously, a comprehensive <u>prescribing history</u> within an EP system is important for ensuring evidence-based working practices and user confidence in the system. However, when the system is designed to provide an optimally comprehensive prescribing record, there are complications associated with the actual transfer of high-granularity prescription data between systems. While transfer of data may be relatively uncomplicated within a system in a physical or wireless networked environment, or through <u>interfaces</u> with other systems in the same hospital location, there are issues associated with transferring data to external systems. There is, for example, currently no model in the UK for transferring medicines data from hospital EP systems – where they exist – to <u>GP systems</u> or <u>community pharmacy systems</u> in <u>primary care</u>.

This is a key driver for <u>regional or national healthcare IT programs</u>, where prescription information is transferred to a central spine, from which it may be retrieved by other healthcare providers as the need arises. Apart from technical issues concerning architecture and hardware, standards for interoperability are required for data formats and messaging. With healthcare application data entities and structures, the international messaging standards are the <u>Health Level 7 (HL7)</u> formats, which are based on XML conventions. For data relating to medicines, the standard terminology is <u>SNOMED CT</u>, from which come the terms for the UK <u>dictionary of medicines and devices (dm±d)</u> [16]. These will be discussed in more detail in the chapter on <u>data support</u> for EP applications. However, at the present time, there is still work to be done on the definition of messages to allow transfer of prescription information between systems at the level of complexity required to support secondary care EP, and also on the ability of applications to receive these messages.

Improvement in Hospital Business Processes Due to Electronic Dissemination of Prescriptions

As mentioned previously, clinical practice in healthcare provider organizations is undertaken in the context of a health economy and practitioners are under pressure to achieve <u>health outcome</u> targets and <u>service level agreements</u>. These pressures exist irrespective of whether the health economy is insurance-driven, as in the US and many countries in continental Europe, or based on central government funding, as with the UK National Health Service. Consequently, healthcare managers in any context are receptive to the use of electronic systems to facilitate greater efficiencies in the use of healthcare resources in a provider organization.

A number of studies have postulated organizational efficiencies as benefits of using an EP system. However, more than perhaps any other EP system benefit area, <u>organizational benefits</u> cited for EP systems are most dependent on the political and socioeconomic contexts in which they are demonstrated. For example, one US study, which reviewed the design of EP software, concluded that detailed system design was important to clinical users and determined how rapidly systems were adopted [17]. The authors concluded that EP design required continuous assessment to ensure relevance to routine practice and user acceptability. This conclusion is consistent with the observation with UK implementations that EP is a "sociotechnical system" and needs to be constantly monitored and developed to deal with unintended consequences of system use in routine healthcare practice [5].

Furthermore, organizational benefits of EP systems are also dependent on the structure and objectives of the study in which they were demonstrated.

Organizational efficiency benefits cited in studies include:

(a) reduced <u>medication ordering turn-around times</u>.
(b) reduced <u>hospital stay times</u>,
(c) streamlining of the <u>hospital discharge</u> process (an important issue in the UK context),
(d) reduced <u>pathology test</u> and <u>radiology test</u> reporting times
(e) reduced number of pathology orders generated, and
(f) improved patient record documentation.

Some studies have indicated that EP has a beneficial effect on <u>medication ordering turnaround times</u>, which is not surprising as many systems facilitate the seamless transmission of prescription data from a prescribing workstation on the ward to a <u>pharmacy system</u> in the pharmacy. One US study has identified a 64% average reduction in <u>medication ordering turn-around time</u> following implementation of an EP system [18]. Another US study [19] looked at the effect of EP systems compared to paper prescribing on dose compliance with first doses of antibiotics. This study found that, with the EP system, there was greater compliance with antibiotic orders, and the medication was delivered to the patient significantly faster than with paper prescribing. A third US study has suggested that EP systems can have a positive effect on the total hospital stay time [20], but this is harder to demonstrate conclusively and may not be replicated in the UK context.

Nevertheless, two of the UK reports indicate that EP is a useful tool for the clinical pharmacist, and helps to streamline the pharmacist's work in terms of the prescription review process, thus allowing them to spend more time on near-patient clinical activities [11, 14].

One important factor in the streamlining of hospital prescribing processes is the ability of the electronic prescribing record to be viewed remotely in a number of different locations

Contribution of Workflow Improvement to Professional Practice Development

Organizational benefits – and in particular, improvement of medicine prescribing, administration and supply workflows within a hospital or healthcare provider organization – have potentially profound implications for the practice of clinical professionals. Due to these efficiencies, healthcare professionals can be confident that time-consuming routine processes can be automated with accuracy, and their time can be released to enable them to engage in more patient-centered activities, which require intuitive input that only a human being can provide. These tasks might include detailed history taking, medicines review, health education, involvement in specialist clinics and patient support groups, clinical research and, of course, evaluating resources and technology that could be used to facilitate further service developments. The staff time that can be released to healthcare professionals following the introduction of an EP system to deal with the routine tasks and processes of hospital prescribing can be significant; one UK study indicated that, in hospitals where there was an EP system, pharmacists could spend up to 70% of their time on activities relating to pharmaceutical care, rather than the prescribing and supply processes [21].

Nevertheless, as well as releasing the time of healthcare professionals to focus on other clinical activities, EP systems provide an infrastructure to support these clinical activities, and to support new and emerging services that can be provided by healthcare professionals. The ways in which EP systems can support professional practice are explored in detail in a subsequent chapter.

Security of Prescriptions and Prescribing Information

As discussed in Chap. 1, the requirement for confidentiality on the part of healthcare professionals is well-established in legislation and in professional standards. The growth of electronic records in healthcare, together with the increased likelihood of electronic dissemination of electronic patient information in local, regional or even national systems beyond the provider institutions has caused health professionals and providers alike to become more concerned about the confidentiality of electronic patient records. The issues relating to confidentiality with electronic systems have most notably been raised with the England NHS Connecting for Health Summary Care Record (SCR) project. For this reasons, health services have become increasingly concerned with requirements for information governance (IG), with electronic systems holding patient information [22]. The information governance agenda covers a range of issues relating to information management and security, and IG requirements will cover the following:

- Appropriate use of passwords or smartcard technology for log in
- Data transfer and encryption
- Security of hardware devices and premises where equipment is used
- Training on confidentiality and management of IG incidents

There are many features in hospital EP systems, which deliver IG and information security requirements. Systems will have password protection, and role-based access, so that users will only have access to the functions of the system that are appropriate to their role. Hospital EP systems will be mounted on dedicated servers and networks, so may be regarded as a closed system, and therefore more secure than traditional paper charts, which are liable to being lost or viewed by unauthorized users.

There are, however, some potential areas of concern. Firstly, the security of wireless networks in different clinical areas should be scrutinized. Secondly, depending on the architecture of the system in terms of the number and type of workstations on each ward, there may specific training requirements for users concerning system security (for both hardware and software access) and data protection. As a rule, the need for information security should be weighed up against the hazards posed by system security arrangements that are too stringent. A simple example of this is that, if the system log on procedure is too complex, users may be tempted to remain logged on at their usual workstation, than to log off between users, which may be counterproductive to information security.

A hospital implementing EP will need to determine how the database of users, their roles and access permissions can be maintained, given the fact that there is often an extensive and high-turnover pool of users (locums, bank staff etc), and that role-based access is an important deliverable for interoperable systems, which is a goal for implementers where there is a regional or national healthcare IT program.

The issue of role based use of systems will be discussed in greater detail in Chap. 6.

Quality of Care Benefits

The reduction of medication errors and improvement in the quality of prescribing are now well-documented benefits of EP systems. The use of the PICS EP system at Birmingham University Hospitals, UK, [23] had a positive impact on quality of care, due to enforcement of local clinical guidance and policies. This included:

- Implementation of the Trust antibiotics policy.
- Daily alert if a patient's prescription does not follow the venous thromboembolism risk assessment guidelines.
- Automatic switching to generic statins for cost reduction, where appropriate.
- Automatic prescribing of methicillin-resistant *Staph. aureus* (MRSA) decolonization medication in patients found to be MRSA positive.

However, there is still little information on whether EP systems have a positive impact on actual patient outcomes, as a result of their influence on clinical practice. One study, by Michelis et al. [24], looked at whether EP use could improve goal attainment in low density lipoprotein (LDL) levels in patients with hyperlipidemia in an outpatient setting. Prescribing records were reviewed retrospectively for an EP system which did not use decision support for hyperlipidemia guideline adherence, but did include formulary decision support, which gave clinicians information about drug costs. Patients receiving electronic prescriptions were 59% more likely to achieve their LDL goal than patients who received paper prescriptions. The authors suggested that this may be because patients whose prescriptions were generated electronically were more likely to receive a generic statin, and this would have a positive impact on optimum dosing.

Further research is required on the impact of EP on actual clinical outcomes, as opposed to healthcare process targets, for various therapeutic areas and public health issues. Nevertheless, there may be difficulties in controlling studies in such a way that a clear causal effect can be seen on a clinical outcome as a result of using an EP system, rather than due to other clinical or environmental factors.

Conclusion

In many organizations where IT has been used to automate business processes, implementers have sought benefits in terms of organizational efficiency, cost-effectiveness and improvements in quality of care. There is emerging evidence that EP systems may have a positive impact on actual clinical outcomes, due to their effects on clinical practice. Further evidence of this is needed, but could be hard to obtain due to the difficulty of designing studies that will adequately control confounding factors. Furthermore benefits observed may be specific to the healthcare context in which they were observed, and may not be reproducible in other health economies. Implementers should consider how existing business processes may be automated, and the extent to which automation may allow new business processes, and support changes in professional roles for, and service development by, health professionals. In order to gain the maximum organizational benefits from EP systems, it is essential that system designers take into account the comments, views and aspirations of clinical users.

References

1. Slee A, Farrar K, et al. Electronic prescribing: implications for hospital pharmacy. Hosp Pharm. 2007;14:217–8.
2. NHS Connecting for Health. Electronic prescribing in hospitals: challenges & lessons learnt. 2009. http://www.connectingforhealth.nhs.uk\systemsandservices\eprescribing. Accessed in October 2010.
3. Kirkman KP. The five foundations of successful E-prescribing programs. Health Manag Technol. 2005; April:32–3.
4. Shane R. Computerised physician order entry: challenges and opportunities. Am J Health Syst Pharm. 2002;59:286–8.
5. Barber N. Electronic prescribing – safer, faster, better? J Health Serv Res Policy. 2010;15 Suppl 1:64–7.
6. Goundrey-Smith SJ. Electronic prescribing – experience in the UK and system design issues. Pharm J. 2006;277:485–9.
7. Gray S, Smith J. Practice report – electronic prescribing in Bristol. Healthc Pharm. 2004; August:20–2.
8. Farrar K. In: Smith J, editor. Building a safer NHS for patients: improving medication safety. London: Department of Health; 2004.
9. Connor AJ, Hutton P, Severn P, Masri I. Electronic prescribing and prescription design in ophthalmic practice. Eur J Ophthalmol. 2011;21:644–8.
10. Farrar K. Accountability, prescribing and hospital pharmacy in an electronic automated age. Pharm J. 1999;263:496–501.
11. Curtis C, Ford NG. Paperless electronic prescribing in a district general hospital. Pharm J. 1997;259:734–5.
12. Fowlie F, Bennie M, Jardine G, Bicknell S, Toner D, Caldwell M. Evaluation of an electronic prescribing and administration system in a British hospital. Pharm J. 2000;265(Suppl):R16.
13. Palchuk MB, Fang EA, et al. An unintended consequence of electronic prescriptions: prevalence and impact of internal discrepancies. J Am Med Inform Assoc. 2010;17:472–6.
14. Foot R, Taylor L. Electronic prescribing and patient records – getting the balance right. Pharm J. 2005;274:210–2.
15. Desroches CM, Agarwal R, Angst CM, Fischer MA. Differences between integrated and stand-alone E-prescribing systems have implications for future use. Health Aff. 2010;29:2268–77.
16. Frosdick P, Dalton C. What is the dm + d and what will it mean for you and pharmacy practice? Pharm J. 2004;273:199–200.
17. Khajouei R, Jaspers MW. The impact of CPOE medication systems' design aspects on usability, workflow and medication orders: a systematic review. Methods Inf Med. 2010;49:3–19.
18. Spencer DC, Leininger A, et al. Effect of a computerised prescriber order entry system on reported medication errors. Am J Health Syst Pharm. 2005;62:416–9.
19. Cunningham TR, Geller ES, Clarke SW. Impact of electronic prescribing in a hospital setting: a process-focused evaluation. Int J Med Inform. 2008;77:546–54.
20. Bates DW, Leape L, et al. Effect of computerised physician order entry and a team intervention on prevention of serious medication errors. J Am Med Assoc. 1998;280:1311–6.
21. Abu Zayed L, Farrar K, et al. An evaluation of drug supply as a component of ward pharmacy activity. Pharm J. 2000;265(Suppl):R68.
22. Goundrey-Smith SJ. Ensure your IT systems are compliant by March. Pharm J. 2011;286:40.
23. Slee A. E-prescribing in Birmingham. Presented at the Guild of Healthcare Pharmacists/ United Kingdom Clinical Pharmacy Association Information Technology Interest Group (ITIG) seminar. Birmingham, UK. 2010. http://www.ghp.org.uk/ContentFiles/ghpitig10a.pps
24. Michelis KC, Hassouna B, et al. Effect of electronic prescription on attainment of cholesterol goals. Clin Cardiol. 2011;34:254–60.

Chapter 4
EP Systems as a Risk Management Tool

The practice of medicine is an inherently risky activity. It is to be hoped that many therapeutic interventions are beneficial when used in the appropriate clinical situation. However, the majority of medical treatment interventions – and indeed some diagnostic or monitoring interventions – carry with them an element of risk. An important aspect of the healthcare professional's job is risk management – to evaluate the risks associated with any particular therapeutic or diagnostic intervention and to follow working practices that reduce the risks involved. The clinical professional evaluates risk on the basis of documented evidence, together with clinical judgment, arising from his or her own professional experience.

Electronic systems cannot completely eradicate risk in medicine since, by definition, they operate heuristically using defined and discreet datasets and logical algorithms, and their ability to be intuitive is limited. Nor can electronic systems address the human elements of the communication of risk information to, and the assimilation of risk information by individual patients. Although electronic systems can provide some information support for this, this aspect of risk assessment remains primarily in the domain of the face-to-face consultation between patient and professional, and rightly so. Nevertheless, there is a reasonable body of evidence to suggest that electronic prescribing systems can reduce prescribing risks that are associated with, or may be influenced by, prescribing procedures.

This chapter will discuss the ways in which EP systems can influence risks associated with the prescribing, supply and medicines administration process. Firstly, however, it is necessary to review the potential risks associated with the medicines management process, and the general principles of how these risks can be managed, before examining specific aspects of risk reduction with EP systems.

Principles of Risk Management in Therapeutics

The medical risks associated with pharmacological therapeutics may be divided into two broad categories:

S. Goundrey-Smith, *Principles of Electronic Prescribing*, Health Informatics,
DOI 10.1007/978-1-4471-4045-0_4, © Springer-Verlag London 2012

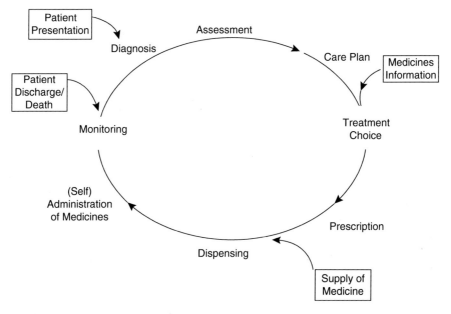

Fig. 4.1 The medicines management cycle

(a) The risks associated with choosing the correct medicine, in the correct formulation and at the correct dose for a particular patient, and

(b) The risks associated with ensuring that, once the correct medicine is chosen for the patient, the correct medicine is then supplied to the patient and that the patient is concordant with treatment.[1]

Figure 4.1 shows the <u>medicines management cycle</u>, a flow diagram for the treatment of a patient with medicines.

As can be seen, the cyclical element to this process is that, depending on the response of a patient to a medicine, the patient may be reassessed, or even re-diagnosed, and the prescribing cycle starts again, with new medicine(s) prescribed instead of, or in addition to, the original prescription.

There are risks associated with each stage in the cycle, and they are as follows:

- <u>Diagnosis</u> – there may be a risk of misdiagnosis, depending on the complexity of the disease, and the probability of atypical presentations. This risk could be reduced with computer <u>decision support</u> tools, or by seeking a specialist second opinion.
- <u>Assessment</u> – disease assessment may be complicated by the use of different scoring or <u>disease activity tools</u> in certain therapeutic areas, and this may lead to

---

[1] *Concordance* is the principle of a patient taking a course of treatment. Concordance is distinct from the notion of *compliance*, which suggests that the patient takes the treatment in order to follow the clinician's instructions and without full commitment to the beneficial possibilities of the treatment.

an inappropriate assessment of a patient's disease. Again, electronic decision support tools may facilitate the appropriate use and interpretation of disease assessment schemas

- Care Plan – lack of <u>clinical guidelines</u>, or guideline interpretation, may mean that individual healthcare providers may not have robust <u>care plans</u> to help clinicians manage different <u>patient groups</u>. In this situation, individual treatment decisions made by clinicians may differ from <u>best practice</u> evidence, thus introducing risks to the patient.

- Choice of Medicine – due to the plethora of pharmacological treatments available, together with their respective <u>efficacy profiles</u>, their <u>contraindications</u> and their <u>licensed uses</u>, the choice of medicine for a patient represents a huge area of risk in the <u>prescribing process</u>. This risk may be compounded by the promotional messages of the <u>pharmaceutical industry</u>, which may not be consonant with established guidance from national prescribing bodies and medical associations. The use of <u>decision support</u> tools in EP has considerable potential to reduce the risks associated with medicine selection, and much research has been conducted into the use of <u>decision support</u> systems to support rational choices of medical treatment. This will be reviewed later in the chapter.

- Prescribing – the prescription written by the prescriber should clearly state the <u>medicine</u>, the <u>formulation</u>, the <u>dose</u>, the <u>route</u>, the <u>frequency</u> and any other special instructions concerning the use of the medicine. When prescriptions are handwritten on hospital <u>drug charts</u>, it is easy for some aspects of the prescription to be unclear or omitted. What often happens in practice in this situation is that the pharmacist will either contact the prescriber to clarify the exact instructions, or may themselves add the necessary additional instructions, if they are satisfied with the prescriber's intention. However, there are risks associated with both of these practices. Furthermore, there is the risk that items may be erroneously omitted or duplicated when a drug chart is rewritten, which can happen at least once during a patient's hospital stay (more often if they are on an acute medical setting, and taking a large number of frequently-changing medicines). Once the prescription is written on the chart, the item has to be obtained either from the pharmacy (often via the hospital's portering system) or selected from the <u>ward stock</u>. Hospital pharmacy staff will be familiar with the perennial problem of lost drug charts or medicines. Electronic prescribing systems have a pivotal role in managing these risks. They can contribute significantly to the completeness and accuracy of prescribing by providing a structured prescribing record for each patient, where all of the prescription data elements are present, together with what might be prescribed as "<u>forcing functions</u>" [1], which ensure that prescribers complete all required entries in the electronic prescription form. Furthermore, an EP system with an electronic link to pharmacy, as discussed in the previous chapter, is able to reduce the risk of the medicine not being present in the clinical area when the patient needs it.

- Dispensing – the risks associated with the dispensing of the medicine are concerning incorrect product selection, and incorrect product <u>labeling</u>. Historically, these risks have existed because the entry of prescriptions onto the <u>pharmacy</u>

system, and the dispensing and labeling of medicines have been manual processes, and have been subject to the human error that can arise in repetitive processes. There is also the risk that treatment cannot go ahead due to medicine supply failure, i.e. the medicine cannot be sourced from the pharmaceutical wholesaler, and an alternative prescription is not facilitated in a timely manner. Where they are being implemented, EP systems are increasingly being interfaced with pharmacy systems and pharmacy robots, thus reducing potential risks in the dispensing process. The issues associated with using EP functionality to manage the supply chain were discussed in some detail in Chap. 3.

• Medicine Administration – traditionally, medicines for hospital inpatients have been administered to each patient from a drug trolley on the ward, according to the instructions on the drug chart (see Chap. 3). The procedure is that the nurse will sign the relevant box on the patient's drug chart to signify that the drug has been given, or put a missed dose code, to show a reason for non-administration, in the box. For Schedule 2 or 3 Controlled Drugs (see Chap. 1), a double check is required before the dose is administered. There are many risks that can arise from the medicine administration process in this form: (a) the incorrect medicine can be supplied from the drug trolley; (b) the correct medicine can be supplied but incorrect details recorded on the drug chart; (c) the patient may receive a time-critical medication late, due to delays in the drug round procedure. The increasing trend towards self-administration of medicines in hospitals may reduce these various sources of error, as patients who are able to self-administer will be familiar with their own regimens. However. EP systems may reduce the risks associated with the medicines administration process, by providing electronic medicines administration, thus making a "closed loop" process (i.e. the whole medicine supply process is controlled electronically), as discussed in the previous chapter. This will reduce risks by providing a clear electronic drug chart, and providing prompts to ensure that each medicine administration event is recorded in a timely fashion.

• Monitoring – in hospital practice, where patients may be critically ill, or who may be having various changes to their medication, monitoring of response to therapy is especially important. EP systems are able to alert clinicians to routine time-dependent monitoring requirements, and can be designed to manage corollary orders, i.e. orders that are raised only in association with other orders. For example, when a patient who is taking potassium-sparing diuretics is then prescribed an ACE inhibitor for heart failure or high blood pressure, their plasma potassium level should be monitored, as the two medicines have an additive effect on potassium levels.

There are a number of general principles of risk management that emerge from a study of the medication management process.

(a) Human error, or operator error where the process is being facilitated by electronic systems, is a major risk element in the prescribing process, since, at various points in the medicines management cycle, human actions and decisions are required. The potential for human error increases when tasks are repetitive or inherently boring. EP systems have the potential to automate tasks in the prescribing process that are repetitive, iterative or which are complex, but predictable, thus minimizing human error in these areas.

(b) Medication errors are often multi-factorial in their causation. To give a simplistic example: a patient is prescribed Amitriptyline 10 mg tablets, and the directions are 1–2 at night. The hyphen on the drug chart becomes illegible, and the patient is given 12 amitriptyline 10 mg tablets in error. In this situation, there are three potential factors which gave rise to this incident. Firstly, the prescriber's instructions were not completely unambiguous; secondly, the pharmacist did not clarify the directions and, thirdly, the nurse administered the dose without querying it. Situations of this nature commonly arise in busy clinical environments and the likelihood of such errors increases with workload, if systems are not in place to monitor the medicines management process. Furthermore, if just one of these factors had been addressed, the incident would not have happened. This phenomenon has been described in medicines risk studies as the so-called "Swiss cheese effect" [2] – i.e. the skewer can pass right through the middle of the cheese, if all the holes line up. Furthermore, at a statistical level, a number of different types of error may contribute to the overall medication error rate in a hospital. These are the sort of statistics that are assessed in qualitative studies of EP systems, which will be reviewed in the remainder of this chapter.

(c) As a general rule, the incidence of medication errors may be reduced by having standard operating procedures (SOPs) in place, which anticipate likely causes of errors, and which reduce any variations in working practice arising from exceptional circumstances. These should closely reflect, and aim to standardize, normative working practice. Each step may be straightforward and even self-explanatory, but documentation of the procedure helps members of staff to follow it, so that it becomes instinctive for them. An example of this is the checking of a patient's hospital number as well as their name, prior to administering drugs.

Reduction in Medication Error Rates with EP Systems: Experience from US Implementations

The potential for an electronic prescribing system to reduce medication errors in hospitals is a key benefit of using the system, given the financial cost of medication errors, both in terms of patient morbidity/mortality and in terms of costs to the healthcare system, both in terms of cost of care and cost of litigation. For this reason, considerable research has been conducted into the extent to which EP systems can reduce medication errors, particularly in the US, where the practice of medicine is highly litigious.

In US studies, reduction in medication errors following the introduction of EP systems is well-documented. In a key US study from the Brigham and Women's Hospital, Boston, Mass., Bates et al. [3] compared computerized physician order entry (CPOE), with CPOE plus a team intervention approach, in the prevention of non-intercepted serious medication errors. They found that, with both interventions, during the implementation period, there was a reduction of non-intercepted serious medication errors by 55%, from 10.7 events per 1,000 patient-days to 4.86 events per 1,000 patient-days (p=0.1). Also, there was a reduction of preventable adverse drug events (ADEs) by 17% (from 4.69 to 3.88 events per 1,000 patient-days), and a reduction of non-intercepted potential adverse drug events (ADEs) by 84% (from 5.99 to 0.98 events per 1,000 patient-days). There was found to be no additional benefit of CPOE plus the team intervention over CPOE alone. The error rate reduction figures of 55% and 84% in this study are substantial, and look impressive, but it must be borne in mind that these figures are for *potential* (non-intercepted) errors, rather than *actual* errors, and it is not clear how many of these potential errors would have become actual errors in practice. The reduction figure for preventable adverse events, 17%, is considerably smaller.

In a follow-up study, Bates et al. [4] looked at medication errors detected in all patients admitted to three medical wards for a 7–10 week periods in four different years (four points in the implementation process). This study took a broader approach than their previous study, in that it looked across the EP implementation period, and that it looked at the effect of CPOE on all error types, not just serious errors. Data were collected at four points in the implementation period:

(a) Period 1 (1992) – at baseline, before EP implementation
(b) Period 2 (1993) – EP system implemented
(c) Period 3 (1995) – allergy checking improved
(d) Period 4 (1997) – drug interaction checking and potassium ordering improved

The ADEs were assessed by pharmacists in a structured manner. The study showed that the overall non missed dose medication error rate decreased by 81%, from 142 ADEs per 1,000 patient-days, to 26.6 ADEs per 1,000 patient-days (p<0.0001). Also, the rate of non-intercepted serious medication errors was reduced by 86% from baseline to period 3 in the implementation process. However, as discussed, since non-intercepted medication errors are by definition those which are not readily detected under normal circumstances, it is difficult to ascertain whether this reduction was as a result of introducing the EP system. Furthermore, this study also showed that the non missed dose error rate actually increased from period 1 to period 2, despite the overall decrease. The study also showed that the missed dose error rate increased between baseline and period 3, and that the intercepted potential ADE rate increased between the baseline interval and period 2. Again, however, the rise in this latter parameter may not be significant since potential errors may not immediately translate into actual errors.

A US baseline analysis of medication errors [5], involving pharmacist evaluation of 1,111 prescribing errors over a week period, indicated that a significant proportion of these (64.4%) could be prevented by EP implementation, and that a further proportion (22.4%) could possibly be prevented, depending on EP system design.

Stone et al. [6] studied error rates with an EP system pre- and post-implementation in an academic surgical unit. They found a very modest level of error reduction; the pre-implementation error rate was 0.22%, the rate of errors in the first 6 months after implementation was 0.16%, which rose to 0.21% after a further 6 months. The fact that this error rate was low and minimally affected by EP implementation may be due to the lack of complex medical regimens in a surgical unit, or because the baseline procedures at the unit were robust. The authors concluded that, while EP systems improved efficiency, they would need to be refined in order to obtain more significant patient safety benefits.

A particular issue with US data on risk reduction with EP systems is the concerning the transcription process. In the US, it is standard practice for hospital staff to produce a drug chart from the physician's clerking notes, and this process is a significant source of medication error in the US setting; some 11% of errors are as a result of the transcription process. Bates et al. [3] indicated that the rate of non-intercepted errors arising from the transcription process was reduced considerably by 84%, from 1.3 events/1,000 patient days to 0.2 events/1,000 patient days. Nebeker et al. [7] also commented that the introduction of CPOE, combined with an electronic medication record, had the potential to obviate the need to transcribe orders, and therefore eliminate transcriptions errors. Such a reduction might be expected if an automated system in being used for electronic dissemination of prescriptions to the hospital pharmacy.

Reduction in Medication Error Rates with EP Systems: Experience from UK Implementations

Fewer United Kingdom centers have published detailed quantitative studies on risk reductions following EP implementation. Furthermore, it is recognized that, since the healthcare system is different in the UK, the risk profile will be different from the US context. Nevertheless, the incidence of medication errors in the UK has been documented. An analysis of medication errors as part of an assessment of a pharmacy intervention scheme [8], indicated baseline incidence rates of 10.1% for medicine administration errors, 6.3% for non-formulary prescribing and 4.6% for transcription errors. All of these could be reduced by implementation of an EP; again, the transcription error rate could be largely eradicated.

Reductions of errors associated with the prescribing process itself have been noted for some UK EP implementations. Farrar [9] has indicated an increase in the number of complete and correct doses on drug charts, following the introduction of EP. In research information available from the Wirral Trust [10], 2,180 prescriptions for 267 patients were analyzed for legibility and completeness, with reference to hospital standards for prescription writing, based on the British National Formulary. Thousand two hundred and seventeen prescriptions generated prior to computerization and 963 prescriptions generated after computerization were assessed; electronic prescribing significantly improved the legibility and completeness of prescriptions, compared to prescribing by hand (p<0.0001).

In a review of EP experience at Wirral, presented at the British Pharmaceutical Conference in 1999 [9], Farrar indicated that the use of EP at the Wirral Hospitals had increased the number of complete and correct doses on drug charts from 17.7% to approaching 100%. However, the record of medicine administration was not always complete; often once only medicines were completely and correctly prescribed, but no record was made of when they were administered.

These improvements in prescription accuracy, and legibility and completeness of prescriptions may be attributed to a number of factors: the availability of a comprehensive drug dataset to support prescribing, and a structured prescribing workflow, and also to the availability to implicit or explicit electronic decision support tools at the point of prescribing.

In their EP implementation in Ayrshire, Scotland, UK, Fowlie et al. [11] noted a significant reduction in inpatient prescribing errors, and medication administration errors, but a non significant reduction in discharge prescribing errors, following the introduction of an EP system. Their main findings were as follows:

1. the EP system led to a significant reduction in the prescribing error rate for inpatient prescriptions but, interestingly, not for discharge prescriptions. The inpatient prescribing error rate fell from 7.4% prior to EP implementation, to 7% 1 month after implementation and then to 4.7% 12 months after implementation (p<0.001). The decrease in prescribing errors with discharge prescriptions, from 7.5% prior to implementation, to 5.9% 12 months after implementation, with an initial increase in error rate to 7.7% after the first month of EP, did not achieve significance.
2. the EP system led to a significant reduction in medication administration errors, from 9% prior to implementation, to 6% 1 month after implementation, and then 5.4% 12 months after implementation (p<0.001). However, medication administration errors involving intravenous drugs and controlled drugs were omitted from these figures, which could affect the overall medication administration error rate.

The observation that the inpatient prescribing error rate was reduced significantly, but the discharge prescribing error rate was not, may reflect the fact that the discharge prescribing process is innately more structured than the inpatient prescribing process, and therefore the potential for error reduction is greater with the inpatient prescribing process. These authors also showed a significant reduction in medicines administration errors, but indicated that the administration of controlled drugs and intravenous drugs were excluded from this assessment. Inclusion of these groups of medicines, and also implementation of the system in an acute medical area, could both adversely affect the outcome concerning medicines administration errors, due to more complex medicines administration scenarios. Consideration should be given to the design of controlled drug prescribing and administration functions, and also to design of functions for prescribing and administration of continuous infusions and other complex intravenous drug regimens. The latter is particularly complicated, in terms of developing clear user interfaces that support all possible prescribing scenarios, and poor design in this area will lead to the introduction of new errors, resulting in critical incidents.

Shulman and colleagues [12] compared the use of a commercial EP system, without decision support functions, with handwritten prescriptions on an intensive care unit at University College Hospital, London, UK. The study found a moderate reduction of medication errors with the EP system. The medication error rate was 6.7% (69 errors on 1,036 prescriptions) for handwritten prescriptions and 4.8% (117 errors on 2,429 prescriptions) for EP generated prescriptions (p<0.04). In addition, there was evidence that error rates with the EP system decreased gradually following its implementation, due to increasing staff familiarity with the system. When both non-intercepted and intercepted errors were combined, patient outcome scores improved under the EP system. However, the three most serious errors that were identified in this study were with the EP system. While it is clear that EP systems can reduce routine errors, they can lead to facilitation of errors, depending on their design.

Charing Cross Hospital, London, UK , has implemented an commercial EP system (ServeRx, MDG Medical, Israel), which deals with all aspects of medicines management in the hospital environment, including electronic medicines administration, with patient identification using barcode technology, and automated dispensing [13]. The system therefore provides a so-called "closed loop" process, in that it automates all aspects of the medicines management process. The system had a positive effect on both medicine prescribing errors and medicine administration errors. The prescribing error rate fell from 3.8% (across 2,450 medicine orders) before EP system implementation, to 2% (across 2,353 orders) after implementation (p<0.001). Non-intravenous medicine administration errors were reduced from 7% (across 1,473 non i/v orders) before the implementation, to 4.3% (across 1,139 orders) after implementation of the system. However, while the system reduced nurse time spent on the medicine administration process, it increased time spent by physicians ordering medicines, and also the time spent by pharmacy staff in providing the ward pharmacy service. The impact of EP systems on the time management of health professionals, and therefore on their patterns of professional practice, is discussed fully in Chap. 6.

In a study conducted at the Sunderland Hospitals, Beard and Candlish [14] note that current UK hospital "kardex" systems are probably unacceptable from a risk perspective, and may exceed the UK Health & Safety Executive's threshold of 1 in 10,000 medication errors per year, although there is no specific evidence to show this. The authors indicated that international research had shown that an automated unit-dose drug distribution system was most likely the safest hospital system. On the basis of this research, together with information on error rates at the Sunderland Hospitals, the authors concluded that if such a system were installed at Sunderland, the system was likely to pay for its investment, in terms of harm reduction, within 2–3 years, and that it would be a positive enhancement to clinical governance. Based on published data and in the

Table 4.1   Risk reduction and cost benefit figures with different elements of electronic medicines management

	Electronic prescribing (CPOE only)	Transcription	Dispensing	Medicines administration
Risk reduction	56%	6%	4% (base line rate at Sunderland – approx 0.05%)	34%
Cost benefit of risk reduction (harm reduction)	£120k pa	£7k pa	£5k pa	£84k pa

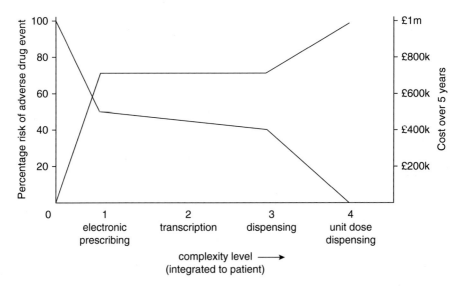

Fig. 4.2 Graph of complexity level of EP system against error reduction and financial cost (Reproduced from Beard and Candlish [14])

context of the Sunderland Hospitals, the authors calculated the following risk reduction figures (Table 4.1):

However, the authors noted that, while greater risk reductions could be obtained with systems of increasing complexity, there was a trade-off against the cost of the system. While a unit dose medicines administration system would be the most effective way of reducing error rates, it would be a considerably bigger investment (Fig. 4.2).

However, the problem with this analysis is that, firstly, it does not take into account the proportion of different types of medication errors that might occur in a specific hospital, and, secondly, the way that different systems may introduce new, unrecognized error types, depending on their configuration. This latter issue will be addressed later in this chapter.

However, EP systems do not completely eradicate medication errors. Abdel Qader et al. [15] studied the use of an EP system in a UK hospital in a 4-week retrospective study. They found that, of 7,920 medication orders for 1,038 patients, 664 (8.4%) were associated with prescribing errors. Omission of drug (31%), incorrect selection of drug (29.4%) and dose regimen errors (18.1%) accounted for most of the errors. Of the 664 errors, 131 (20.8%) were considered minor, 481 (76.3%) were considered significant and 18 (2.9%) were considered serious. The authors concluded that prescribing errors can occur at discharge even with the intervention of an EP system. However, the EP system facilitated the systematic extraction of data to enable analysis of prescribing errors. In this way, the EP system can serve as a tool to identify all kinds of prescribing error, even those that would not be prevented by an EP system.

Reduction in Medication Error Rates with EP Systems: Experience from Implementations in Europe

Quantitative studies on the operation of EP systems have also been published by centers in Europe. Van Doormaal et al. [16] studied the effect of an EP system with clinical decision support on the incidence of medication errors and adverse drug events (ADEs) in a hospital in the Netherlands. They found that the percentage of medication orders containing at least one error dropped from 55% prior to implementation of the EP system to 17% post-implementation. While there was also a reduction of ADEs in the hospital after implementation of the EP system, a causal link between the two could not be demonstrated, because of the interrupted time-series design of the study.

In a quantitative evaluation of an EP system in Switzerland, Bonnabry et al. [17] noted that the patient safety benefits of the EP system were dependent on the exact EP functions implemented, and how easy they are for the user to operate. This finding correlates well with Barber's observation that EP systems are not "plug and play" systems, but sociotechnical systems, where the safety of the whole system depends on the interaction of the human operator as well as the operation of the computer [18].

Effect of EP Systems on Medication Error Rates in Pediatrics

Pediatrics is a high risk medical specialty in terms of therapeutics, due to low doses of medicines, complex dosing schedules based on body weight or surface area, drugs being used with a narrow therapeutic index, and non-standard, age related pharmacokinetics of certain drugs. It is likely then that appropriate EP systems could have a beneficial effect on medication error rates in pediatric settings, and a number of studies have been published in this specialty. In a study of pediatric prescribing in five UK hospitals, Ghaleb et al. [19] concluded that EP systems have the potential to reduce dosing errors and errors relating to missing information, but that EP systems would not be rapidly adopted in the pediatric setting. These findings are reflected in the available quantitative studies on pediatric EP at the current time.

Jani et al. [20] studied the use of an EP system in renal patients at a pediatric hospital. The overall error rate was 77.4% with handwritten prescriptions, which was reduced to 4.8% following introduction of the EP system. Many of the errors prior to EP implementation were related to important information omitted from the prescription (73.5%); these errors of omission were most likely reduced by prompts in the EP workflow, when the system was in operation.

Warwick et al. [21] audited prescribing errors and omitted doses before and after EP implementation in a pediatric intensive care unit. They found that the prescribing error rate decreased from 8.8% prior to implementation to 8.1% 1 week after implementation (a non significant reduction), and then to 4.6% 6 months after implementation. Omitted doses were reduced significantly from 8.1% before implementation, to 1.6% 6 months after implementation, albeit with a rise to 10.6% in the week immediately following implementation.

Kazemi et al. [22] studied the error rate for an EP system in a pediatric environment, comparing intervals of physician order entry (POE) and nurse order entry (NOE). They found that prescribing errors decreased from 10.3% during POE to 4.6% during the NOE period, and compliance with warnings was 44% for POE and 68% with NOE. These results suggest that nurse involvement in the EP process reduced error rates and improved compliance and that, if physicians are resistant to EP implementation, nurse use of the system might facilitate the implementation process.

A US study [23] compared the number of adverse events during 1,200 pediatric hospital admissions, before and after installation of an EP system. Seventy-six and 94 adverse events occurred before implementation, compared to 37 and 35 after implementation, a significant decrease. The system was most effective at reducing adverse events associated with prescribing of aminoglycosides and cephalosporins. The authors concluded that an EP system with comprehensive decision support functions reduced errors associated with pediatric hospital admissions, but that refinements were required to gain further safety benefits.

Jani et al. [24] studied the use of a commercial EP system at a tertiary care children's hospital in the UK. They found that, prior to EP implementation, prescribing errors occurred in 88 of 3,929 items prescribed (2.2%), and in 57 of 4,784 items prescribed (1.2%) after implementation. A decrease in the severity rating of errors was also noted after EP implementation. The authors concluded that, while EP appeared to reduce medication errors in the pediatric setting, larger studies were required to assess the impact of EP on error severity, and in different settings.

Current studies suggest that EP has the potential to reduce risks associated with prescribing specifically in a pediatric patient population, in particular errors associated with omission of prescription information. However, as with EP in general patient populations, further studies are required to assess the impact of EP on prescribing errors in detail.

Role of Barcodes in EP Systems

Automated systems have the potential to reduce errors and manage risk at the supply end of the medicines use process. The UK Audit Commission's "Spoonful of Sugar" report [25], published in 2001, highlighted the potential of pharmacy automation to reduce dispensing error rates. Following on from that report, many hospital pharmacy departments constructed business cases to install automated dispensing systems (pharmacy robots), and to re-engineer pharmacy services. The operational aspects of these, and their relationship with EP systems, have been discussed in the previous chapter. A further study by Beard and Candlish at Sunderland [26] examined the extent to which an EP system could reduce the incidence of dispensing errors. An important general factor is that, because traditional dispensing is a manual process, error rates will to some extent be dependent on the number of staff present in a dispensary, and so dispensing error figures should be adjusted to take this into account, and be expressed as errors per member of staff. The authors found that the use of the EP system for inpatient medicine ordering led to an dispensing error rate of 0.0029 errors per person, compared to 0.0045 – 0.0057 errors per person in other areas of the hospital. One of the pharmacies in the Trust used barcode product selection, which achieved a slightly lower dispensing error rate of 0.0022 errors per person. Due to the high ratio of staff to prescriptions, and the highly controlled environment, the lowest dispensing error rate was in the Trust's chemotherapy manufacturing facility, where the authors calculated an error rate of zero.

Barcode technology has also been used by EP systems in order to reduce errors in the medication administration process on the ward. The patient's wristband barcode is scanned prior to a medicine administration event to confirm patient identity, and the barcode on the medicine is scanned to confirm the identity of the medicine to be administered. Medicines administration with the assistance of barcodes to identify either the patient or the drug may contribute to reductions in levels of medicine administration errors at the point of administration. In the Charing Cross study [13], the EP system process forced nurses to use the barcode system for patient identification, and the percentage of patients who were not definitively identified prior to medicines administration decreased from 82.6% before EP system implementation, to 18.9% after system implementation.

The limitations with use of barcodes are the availability, configuration and scalability of appropriate hardware, and also the fact that there is a proportion of medicines that do not have a correct barcode identifier. The use of barcodes may also be limited by harmonization issues and obsolescence, due to development of RFID (radio frequency identification) technology [27]. In addition, use of barcodes for reduction of medicine administration errors relies on use of original packs (with barcodes) at ward level in a hospital.

Increases in Medication Errors Due to the Introduction of EP Systems

An important finding in some US studies is that the implementation of an EP system can actually increase the number of medication errors reported, at least at the outset. In the first of these studies, the Bates 1999 study [4], an increase in error rate was noted during the initial stages of the study, as noted earlier. The increase in error rate was attributed to the EP system's functionality for dealing with potassium orders, which was only finalized later in the implementation process. In the second study, an observational review of a CPOE implementation at the University of North Carolina Hospitals [28], the increase in medication error rate was attributed to (a) increased ability to identify errors due to enhanced data capture on an electronic system, (b) errors generated by staff unfamiliar with a new system, or (c) error detection bias (due to either pre-conceived ideas about EP by users, or evaluators keen to report errors in a new system).

More worryingly, it has been suggested in some studies that the very design of EP systems could facilitate errors, leading to hitherto uncharacterized errors. Koppel et al. [29] did a study of medication errors generated by a commercial EP system that had been in operation in a US hospital for 7 years. They found that the EP system facilitated 22 error types, which fell into two groups: (a) errors generated by the fragmentation of data by the system and lack of integration between the different components of the system, (b) errors arising from the human-machine interface.

Nebeker et al. [7] commented on how a high rate of adverse drug events (ADEs) could occur even at a hospital where there was a high level of IT usage, to support hospital processes. The study looked at ADEs across the electronic prescribing process, by performing a prospective daily review of the electronic medical record for a random sample of all admissions over a 20 week period at a US hospital. The study showed that, of 937 admissions, there were significant ADEs in 483 admissions. 99% of the ADEs identified resulted in serious harm to the patient, and 27% of the ADEs were due to medication. The study observed that ADE rates were still relatively high after CPOE introduction, if decision support systems are not present as an integral part of the system. The role of decision support systems in reducing prescribing risk with electronic systems is discussed in detail in the next section.

This phenomenon has also been noted in the UK. As mentioned previously in this chapter, an initial increase in prescribing error rate following implementation of EP (leading to an eventual reduction in error rate), was demonstrated at the Ayrshire and Arran Trust, Scotland [11], for discharge prescriptions, and this observation was responsible for the reduction of prescribing error rate for discharge prescriptions not reaching overall statistical significance. This effect was also noted in the comparative study of an EP system with handwritten prescriptions in the intensive care unit context [12], where the three major errors occurred with the EP system. The authors concluded that clinicians should not become complacent about the use of automated systems to eradicate errors.

A number of subsequent studies have identified the potential for EP systems to generate new errors that would not have occurred prior to use of the system. Flebbe et al. [30] examined the use of an EP system on an orthopedic surgery ward in a Danish hospital. They found that the EP system could generate new types of error, and that some of these errors could be prevented by improvements in the user interface/workflow, and user training.

Magrabi et al. [31] examined prescribing practice with an EP system in a cohort of hospital doctors under laboratory conditions, to assess the errors that EP system operation could introduce. In the study, 32 doctors completed four tasks, with planned interruptions, and across the four prescribing tasks, an error rate of between 0.5% and 16% was noted; the wide variation is probably due to the small sample size. A range of different errors occurred in the prescribing process – failure to enter allergy information, incorrect medicine selection, incorrect route, dose, formulation and frequency of administration, and omission of start date, administration times and discontinuation date. Unsurprisingly, complex tasks took longer to complete. The authors indicated that prompts in the workflow may have prevented errors due to task interruption, but that more research was required to evaluate the effects of interruption.

Reckmann et al. [32] conducted a review of 13 hospital EP studies published between 1998 and 2007. While nine of the studies demonstrated a significant reduction in prescribing errors, several studies reported errors such as increased rates of duplicate medicines, and failure to discontinue medicines (although these errors types are possible with paper-based prescribing). The authors concluded that the evidence for the safety benefits of EP systems is not compelling and that further research was required using larger sample sizes, more controlled conditions and standard definitions of errors and adverse events. The issues relating to the methodology of EP study design are discussed in more detail later in this chapter.

Reduction of Medication Errors Due to the Availability of Electronic Decision Support Tools at the Point of Prescribing

In the study by Nebeker et al. [7], documenting 937 hospital admissions, it was found that 483 admissions had significant adverse drug events associated with them and that 27% of these were associated with medication. Of the medication-related adverse drug events, 61% were associated with prescribing errors and 25% with monitoring errors and the authors concluded that EP with decision support (DS) features would have a major impact on these error rates, by reducing inappropriate prescribing at the outset, and by providing suitable monitoring tools when certain drugs are prescribed (e.g. digoxin, lithium, theophylline). Indeed, the consensus among electronic prescribing specialists is that decision support tools should be an integral part of EP systems, as they have the potential to "add value" to the system as a clinical tool. The above data suggest that DS functions are particularly valuable in reducing selection errors and inappropriate selection at the medicine ordering stage of the medicines management cycle, and thus reduce risks associated with prescribing errors.

Clinical decision support facilities may be classified into *active* decision support, or *passive* decision support. Active decision support functions provide a clinical alert to the user automatically as part of the workflow of the system, without the user having to actively seek the clinical information. Active decision support mechanisms are built into the EP system software. Passive decision support functions, however, are stand-alone medicines information reference sources mounted on the internet, an intranet or a local server, and accessible via a "hot key" or quick link by a clinical user, when the user is actively seeking information to resolve a clinical problem. Medicines information reference sources which may be incorporated into EP systems will be discussed in Chap. 5.

Clinical decision support warnings and information would include some or all of the following:

(a) sensitivity checking
(b) drug interactions
(c) duplicate therapy/drug doubling
(d) precautions/contraindications
(e) dose checking
(f) formulary status, and
(g) monitoring warnings.

The key issue with active DS functions is that they must be sufficiently comprehensive to be of clinical value, but designed in such a way that they are not excessively presented to the clinical user, which might lead to important warnings being disregarded by the user (warning fatigue). This is a delicate balance and requires considerable thought if the rules are going to be configured within the EP application – for this reason, some implementers have chosen not to support DS functions at all, rather than implement them in a partial manner or without full evaluation; this is the reason why the EP project at Southmead Hospital, Bristol, did not implement any DS functions [33]. In the past, for example, there have been some systems that have limited the number of drug interaction warnings to two or three per drug, or limited the number of allergens for sensitivity checking to two per patient. Limitations of this nature are clearly not acceptable if an EP system is to provide comprehensive DS functions.

However, with a comprehensive DS tool, based on a drug database from a third party data supplier, these issues can be addressed by the mode of implementation of the DS functions in the EP application; with, for example, the use of graded drug interactions, where the system can be configured so that the most clinically significant drug interactions are displayed prominently to clinical users, or flagging of absolute contraindications as a priority. The advantages and disadvantages of using a third party data supplier to enable DS functions will be discussed in the next chapter.

The issue of warning fatigue is well-recognized. On a retrospective analysis of allergy alerts in an EP system, Huntemann et al. [34] found that, out of 49,887 medication orders, 643 orders gave rise to an allergy alert, but that 625 of the 643 alerts

(97%) were overridden, either because the patient had previously tolerated the medication, the benefits outweighed the risk, or for some other reason. The quantitative impact of allergy alerts is therefore low.

Another question to be addressed in the provision of DS is whether there is any type of prescription that should be completely disallowed by a DS function on the EP system – i.e. whether a hard stop should be placed on the prescribing process. There are some prescriptions that are absolutely dangerous and that should (and could) be prevented automatically by an EP system – so-called "never events", for example, intrathecal use of vincristine, daily dosing of methotrexate. The EP system used on the renal unit at the Queen Elizabeth Medical Centre, Birmingham, UK [35] disallowed some orders because of sensitivities and serious drug interactions. However, careful consideration should be given to the issue of disallowing prescriptions because of relative contraindications; if too many prescription types are automatically disallowed, clinicians may choose to bypass the system and write prescriptions by hand, thus defeating the object of an EP system and compromising the completeness of the electronic prescribing record. Strom et al. [36] looked at the use of a hard stop on the co-prescribing of warfarin and co-trimoxazole. They found that, while the alert was highly effective in changing prescribing behavior (i.e. the prescriber had no choice but to abandon the prescription), it led to clinically significant delays in treatment initiation, which caused the termination of the study.

There are also issues concerning the usefulness of decision support algorithms for alerting on contraindications and high doses. In designing a decision support algorithm for contraindications, Ferner and Coleman [37] remarked that many contraindications were due to co-morbidities, and the decision support algorithm was reliant on relevant clinical data being available in the patient's electronic patient record, which was by no means always the case. Seidling et al. [38] designed an algorithm to alert for high doses of some 170 drugs, taking into account age, renal function and contraindications, but the high dose alert was triggered on only 4.5% of prescriptions and that clinicians were responsive to only one in four high dose alerts, either because the alert was inappropriate, or the dose prescribed was, in fact, appropriate for the patient. The value of such an algorithm is therefore questionable if its application is limited and it is so readily overridden by the clinician's judgment.

In any case, if systems provide integral application algorithms for calculations (e.g. renal function, hepatic function, body surface area), rather than using a third-party "black box", then clinical users will need to establish whether these are user configurable and how they will be validated and maintained.

Some authors have indicated that use of an EP system made it easier to monitor prescribing habits within a hospital [9]. It is possible to control choice of formulary medicines over non-formulary medicines by the system either (a) guiding prescribers towards formulary medicines, or (b) disallowing prescription of non formulary medicines. Initially, there was some evidence to suggest that EP systems do not have a major impact on the balance of formulary and non-formulary prescribing [39]. However, a number of studies have been published recently to suggest that EP systems can improve therapeutic guideline compliance [40], increase the rate of generic medicine prescribing with a corresponding decrease in branded medicine prescribing [41], and lead to a sustained increase in the rate of generic medicine prescribing, following implementation [42]. All of these effects could lead to a reduction in costs of care by healthcare providers, although the exact costs – and any unintended consequences – will be dependent on the healthcare context.

DS applications have been in use in the US for some years and, due to their potentially pivotal role in preventing medication errors, they have been subject to a great deal of quantitative research in the US medical literature.

Despite some of the potential problems described above, the benefits of DS systems are well-documented. Teich et al. [43] conducted a time series analysis of an EP system where, as new medication orders are entered, the system displayed drug usage guidelines, including dose and frequency information. The EP system led to various positive changes in prescribing practice. These included (a) an increase in the percentage of orders for the formulary recommended drug in a particular drug class; (b) a decrease in the percentage of orders for a drug with doses that exceeded the recommended maximum dose for that drug, and (c) an increase in the use of the approved frequency of administration for a drug.

Hunt et al. [44] performed a systematic review on 68 controlled studies of prescribing DS systems. The effect of a DS system on physician performance was assessed in 65 of the studies and, in 43 of these studies (66%), a benefit to the physician was demonstrated. A majority of studies demonstrated benefits to the physician for drug dosing systems, preventive care systems and other medical care applications. Physician benefits were not adequately demonstrable for diagnostic DS tools, but the sample size in this review consisted of only five studies. The authors also concluded that further work would be required to assess the impact of DS systems on health outcomes, rather than physician performance.

More recently, there has been a growth in the available literature on specialist applications of decision support and their benefits. The available studies are shown in Table 4.2 below.

In the US, the Joint Clinical Decision Support Workgroup (JCDSWG) has published recommendations for EP system DS function development [56]. The group recognized that the benefits of DS functions used in EP systems had not been fully realized, and that further development of DS systems was required. They reported recommendations and action plans in three general domains:

- advances in system capabilities (DS knowledge base, database elements, usability and performance).
- Standardization and centralization of vocabularies and knowledge structures, so that standard DS routines do not need to be adapted by software vendors and healthcare providers.
- financial and legal incentives to promote adoption of DS within EP systems.

However, research by Wang et al. [57] has shown that, on average, available EP systems in the US fulfill only half of these recommendations. It is this lack of advanced functionality that will need to be addressed before EP systems can have a positive effect on financial cost and health outcomes in chronic diseases in the US; this is one of the issues addressed by the Medicare Modernization Act 2003.

Table 4.2 Quantitative decision support studies

Authors	Setting	Decision support intervention	Key findings	References
Evans et al.	US hospital	Decision support system for antibiotic prescribing (n=545 patients; control=1,136 patients)	Reduction in number of orders for drugs for which patients had known sensitivities (from 146 orders to 35 (p<0.01))	[45]
			Reduction of excessive drug doses (from 405 orders to 87 (p<0.01))	
			Prevention of antibiotic-susceptibility mismatches (reduction from 206 events to 12 (p<0.01))	
			Reduction in the mean number of days of excessive drug doses (from 5.9 days to 2.7 (p<0.002))	
			Reduction in the number of adverse drug events caused by antibiotics (from 28 events to 4 (p<0.02))	
Clemens et al.	US hospital	Insulin guideline for non critically ill Type II diabetes patients	The majority of patients did not receive the preferred insulin regimen probably because the guideline was not incorporated into the prescribing workflow in an interruptive manner	[46]

(continued)

Table 4.2 (continued)

Authors	Setting	Decision support intervention	Key findings	References
Bourgeois et al.	US hospital	Acute respiratory infection treatment template	The template reduced inappropriate antibiotic prescribing for acute respiratory infection in children, but overall use of the template was low, again because it was not incorporated into the prescribing workflow in an interruptive manner	[47]
Papaioannou et al.	Canadian long term care setting	Warfarin monitoring system	Improvement in time to therapeutic range Reduced numbers of INR venepunctures Streamlined prescribing and monitoring processes	[48]
Trafton et al.	US healthcare setting	Decision support for opioid prescribing in chronic pain	Use of an iterative process led to development of a multifunctional DS system which was endorsed by clinical guideline authors, content specialists and clinicians	[49]
Milner et al.	US mental health setting	Decision support for prescribing in schizophrenia, bipolar disorder and depression	Increased compliance to mental health treatment guidelines. Providers were adherent for 32% of their patients in the first 6 months after implementation, and 52% in the second 6 months.	[50]

Tang et al.	Specialist dermatology centre, Singapore	Decision support for isotretinoin prescribing	Increased compliance to isotretinoin prescribing guidance – compliance moved from a baseline of 50–60% to greater than 90% for 30 consecutive months post implementation	[51]
Field et al.	US long term medical setting	Decision support for prescribing in renal patients	Prescribing was more appropriate, and prescribing decisions were of higher quality. Final drug orders were clinically appropriate significantly more often in the intervention group (RR = 1.2 (1.0–1.4))	[52]
Lesprit et al.	French hospital	Decision support system prompting post-prescrition review of antibiotic prescriptions	Reduced number of days of antibiotic therapy in the intervention group (p < 0.0001) Improved quality of antibiotic prescribing. Greater compliance to the recommendations of the attending physician	[53]

(continued)

Table 4.2 (continued)

Authors	Setting	Decision support intervention	Key findings	References
Buising et al.	Australian hospital	Computerized antimicrobial approval system	Appropriate increase in prescriptions for broad spectrum antibiotics Corresponding reduction in 3rd and 4th generation cephalosporins, carbapenems etc. Improved susceptibility of Pseudomonas spp. to many antibiotics No increases in adverse outcomes for patients with Gram negative bacteraemia	[54]
Cooley	US hospital	Venous thromboembolism (VTE) risk calculator	The system reduced the incidence of VTE by 41%. In 2008, 2,050 alerts led to a pharmacist intervention, of which 85% were accepted by medical staff. However, with only 33% of the alerts was prophylaxis actually prescribed.	[55]

In response to these publications, Miller et al. [58], highlighted the ability of large academic medical centers to implement complex EP systems, but that smaller, rural healthcare providers do not have the expertise or financial resources to implement such system. Furthermore, Miller et al. claimed that, while the DS functions of well-established EP systems at centers of excellence are often maintained in house, the third party drug database used in commercial EP systems that would be implemented elsewhere may not be of such high quality. This claim will be examined in more detail in the next chapter on data support. Miller and colleagues argue for the development of US-wide drug database and terminology standards to support DS, and indicated that EP systems would not be implemented widely across the US, in rural areas as well as major conurbations, until that happened.

Problems with Evaluating Risk Reduction Aspects of EP Systems

With many of the quantitative studies described here, whose purpose is to perform a statistical analysis on error rates and other risk issues in the medicines management process, and to evaluate an EP system as an intervention in the process, there are potential confounding factors. These may include the following:

(a) the subjectivity of reviewers in the evaluation of adverse drug events and medication errors in these studies;
(b) the lack of parallel studies between units with EP and those without EP in the same hospital;
(c) the extent to which the study period represents the full implementation schedule of the EP system. If certain functions of an EP system are not available, this may have a profound effect on the error rates detected by a quantitative study.
(d) error detection bias in error reporting, due to the vigilance of researchers and users when evaluating a new system, and
(e) the extent to which the benefits reported are specific to the working practices of the sites studied.

The extent to which these confounding factors associated with research methodology or system design affect benefits needs to be evaluated in more detail.

A number of papers have commented on the methodology of quantitative evaluations of EP systems. In a systematic review, Ammenwerth et al. [59] noted that, while EP systems can reduce the risk of medication errors, quantitative studies varied considerably in their setting, design, quality and results. The authors called for more randomized controlled trial methodology covering a wider range of clinical settings and geographical locations. Similarly, following their review of EP studies, Reckmann et al. [32] called for greater control of EP study conditions, larger sample sizes and standardized definitions of error types.

It has been suggested [60] that there should be a formal methodology for validation of EP software, analogous to the process of licensing a new medicine. However, while a prospective, controlled study is the "gold standard" in clinical medicine, and especially therapeutics, to demonstrate associations and causal links, such studies are much harder to design to assess clinical informatics interventions.

In his discussion of the methodologies for evaluation of EP systems, Trent Rosenbloom [61] describes a number of problems in the design of clinical informatics studies, including (a) the isolations of specific system variables to be tested, (b) the choice of the most appropriate units of study (individual patient, ward, consultant list or hospital) to be exposed to the system variable under study conditions, and (c) ensuring that the study groups remain distinct during the time that systems or workflows are tested, and that there is no inadvertent cross-over of subjects.

While there is a clear need for quantitative data on the operation of EP systems, the insights that qualitative techniques can provide should not be discounted. Savage et al. [62] compared medication error rate pictures obtained by quantitative and qualitative methods at an English hospital after implementation of an EP system. They concluded that, while the two processes provided an similar picture of the drug use process, interviews took less time to conduct than retrospective record review (and were therefore more cost-effective), provided more information on the prescribing process, identified two errors that were not found in record review and provided reasons for delayed or omitted administration of medicines.

Barber et al. [18] reviewed progress with implementation of EP systems, evaluating the implementations at Burton on Trent, and Charing Cross Hospital, London, in the UK. They concluded that, although EP systems reduce medication errors, their implementation is not straightforward, and they should always be regarded as work in progress. Effectiveness of EP systems should be regularly monitored, because of changing human systems and test platforms. Green et al. [63] has commented on the perception in health services that EP systems can eradicate medication errors and reduce the need for clinical pharmacists. The likely situation however is that, given the need for ongoing monitoring of EP systems for effectiveness and emergence of new errors, the need for clinical pharmacy input is likely to remain, if not increase, in order to achieve the lowest possible medication error rates within a hospital.

Conclusion

There is now a large body of research evidence to suggest that EP systems reduce risks associated with the prescribing, administration and supply of medicines. Reduction of prescribing errors has been noted in pediatric settings as well as in general patient populations. Decision support (DS) systems in conjunction with EP systems have been evaluated at length and, while these systems offer many benefits, their use may be limited by lack of supporting data and the fact that they are not integral to the EP workflow. Risk reductions achieved with EP systems are dependent on system design, and the definitions and methodologies of the quantitative studies used to evaluate them. It is also recognized that EP systems can introduce new and hitherto uncharacterized risks to the medicines management process. There is a need for ongoing monitoring of current EP implementations to assess error rates and identify any unintended consequence of system use. There is also a need to evaluate newly implemented EP systems, and devise formal controlled study methodology for this purpose.

References

1. Bates DW, Gawande AA. Improving Safety with Information Technology. N Engl J Med. 2003;348:2525–34.
2. Reason J. Human Error: Models and Management. Br Med J. 2000;320:768–70.
3. Bates DW, Leape L, et al. Effect of Computerised Physician Order Entry and a Team Intervention on Prevention of Serious Medication Errors. J Am Med Assoc. 1998;280:1311–6.
4. Bates DW, Teich JM, et al. The impact of computerised physician order entry on medication error prevention. J Am Med Inform Assoc. 1999;6:313–21.
5. Bobb A, Gleason K, et al. The epidemiology of prescribing errors: the potential impact of computerised physician order entry. Arch Intern Med. 2004;164:785–92.
6. Stone WM, Smith BE, Shaft JD, Nelson RD, Money SR. Impact of a computerised physician order entry system. J Am Coll Surg. 2009;208:960–7.
7. Nebeker J, Hoffman JM, et al. High Rates of Adverse Drug Events in a Highly Computerised Hospital. Arch Intern Med. 2005;165:1111–6.
8. Dodd C. Assessing pharmacy interventions at Salisbury Healthcare NHS Trust. Hosp Pharm. 2003;10:451–6.
9. Farrar K. Accountability, prescribing and hospital pharmacy in an electronic, automated age. Pharm J. 1999;263:496–501.
10. Farrar K. In: Smith J, editor. Building a safer NHS for patients: improving medication safety. London: Department of Health; August 2004.
11. Fowlie F, Bennie M, et al. Evaluation of an electronic prescribing and administration system in a British Hospital. Pharm J. 2000;265(Suppl):R16.
12. Shulman R, Singer M, et al. Medication errors: a prospective cohort study of handwritten and computerised physician order entry in the intensive care unit. Crit Care. 2005;9:R516–21.
13. Franklin BD, O'Grady K, et al. The impact of a closed-loop electronic prescribing and administration system on prescribing errors, administration errors and staff time: a before and after study. Qual Saf Health Care. 2007;16:279–84.
14. Beard R, Candlish C. Does Electronic Prescribing contribute to Clinical Governance? Br J Healthc Comput. 2004;21:27–9.
15. Abdel Qader DH, Harper L, Cantrill JA, Tully MP. Pharmacists' interventions in prescribing errors at hospital discharge: an observational study in the context of an electronic prescribing system in a UK teaching hospital. Drug Saf. 2010;33:1027–44.
16. Van Doormaal JE, van den Bemt PM, et al. The influence that electronic prescribing has on medication errors and preventable adverse drug events: an interrupted time-series study. J Am Med Inform Assoc. 2009;16:816–25.
17. Bonnabry P, Despont-Gros C, et al. A risk analysis method to evaluate the impact of a computerised provider order entry system on patient safety. J Am Med Inform Assoc. 2008;15:453–60.
18. Barber N. Electronic Prescribing – Safer, Faster, Better? J Health Serv Res Policy. 2010;15 Suppl 1:64–7.
19. Ghaleb MA, Barber N, et al. The incidence and nature of prescribing and medication administration errors in paediatric inpatients. Arch Dis Child. 2010;95:113–8.
20. Jani YH, Ghaleb MA, et al. Electronic prescribing reduced prescribing errors in a pediatric renal outpatient clinic. J Pediatr. 2008;152:214–8.

21. Warrick C, Naik H, Avis S, Fletcher P, Franklin BD, Inwald D. A clinical information system reduced medication errors in paediatric intensive care. Intensive Care Med. 2011;37:691–4.
22. Kazemi A, Fors UG, Tofighi S, Tessma M, Ellenius J. Physician order entry or nurse order entry? Comparison of two implementation strategies for computerised order entry system aimed at reducing dosing medication errors. J Med Internet Res. 2010;12:e5.
23. Holdsworth MT, Fichtl RE, et al. Impact of computerized prescriber order entry on the incidence of adverse drug events in pediatric inpatients. Pediatrics. 2007;120:1058–66.
24. Jani YH, Barber N, Wong IC. Paediatric dosing errors before and after electronic prescribing. Qual Saf Health Care. 2010;19:337–40.
25. Audit Commission. A spoonful of sugar – medicines management in NHS hospitals. London: Audit Commission; 2001.
26. Beard R, Candlish C. Is electronic prescribing the best system for preventing pharmacy dispensing errors Br. J Healthc Comput. 2007;24:15–8.
27. Adcock H. European Association of Hospital Pharmacy Congress: RFID raises issues associated with privacy and data collision. Hosp Pharm. 2006;13:138.
28. Spencer DC, Leininger A, et al. Effect of a computerised prescriber order entry system on reported medication errors. Am J Health Syst Pharm. 2005;62:416–9.
29. Koppel R, Metlay JD, et al. Role of computerised physician order entry systems in faciliating medical errors. J Am Med Assoc. 2005;293:1197–203.
30. Flebbe E, Jensen T, Andersen P. Does electronic medicine prescription cause new types of errors? Ugeskr Laeger. 2009;171:2260–4.
31. Magrabi F, Li SY, Day RO, Coiera E. Errors and electronic prescribing; a controlled laboratory study to examine task complexity and interruption effects. J Am Med Inform Assoc. 2010;17:575–83.
32. Reckmann MH, Westbrook JI, Koh Y, Lo C, Day RO. Does computerised provider order entry reduce prescribing errors for hospital inpatients? A systematic review. J Am Med Inform Assoc. 2009;16:613–23.
33. Gray S, Smith J. Practice report – electronic prescribing in Bristol. Healthc Pharm. 2004; August:20–2.
34. Hunteman L, Ward L, et al. Analysis of allergy alerts within a computerised prescriber order entry system. Am J Health Syst Pharm. 2009;66:373–7.
35. Nightingale PG, Adu D, Richards NT, Peters M. Implementation of rules-based computerised bedside prescribing and administration: intervention study. Br Med J. 2000;320:750–3.
36. Strom BL, Schinnar R, Aberra F, Bilker W, Hennessy S, Leonard CE, Pifer E. Unintended effects of a computerised physician order entry nearly hard stop alert to prevent a drug interaction. Arch Intern Med. 2010;170:1578–83.
37. Ferner RE, Coleman JJ. An algorithm for integrating contraindications into electronic prescribing decision support. Drug Saf. 2010;33:1089–96.
38. Seidling HM, Schmitt SP, Bruckner T, Kaltschmidt J, Pruszydlo MG, Senger C, Bertsche T, Walter-Sack I, Haefeli WE. Patient specific electronic decision support reduces prescription of excessive doses. Qual Saf Health Care. 2010;19:E15.
39. Ross SM, Papshev D, Murphy EL, Sternberg DJ, Taylor J, Barg R. Effects of electronic prescribing on formulary compliance and generic drug utilisation in the ambulatory care setting: a retrospective analysis of administrative claims data. J Manag Care Pharm. 2005;11:418–9.
40. Went K, Antoniewicz P, et al. Reducing prescribing errors: can a well-designed electronic system help? J Eval Clin Pract. 2010;16:556–9.
41. Fischer MA, Vogeli C, et al. Effect of electronic prescribing with formulary decision support on medication use and cost. Arch Intern Med. 2008;168:2433–9.
42. Stenner SP, Chen Q, Johnson KB. Impact of generic substitution decision support on electronic prescribing behaviour. J Am Med Inform Assoc. 2010;17:681–8.
43. Teich JM, et al. Effects of computerised physician order entry on prescribing practices. Arch Intern Med. 2000;160(18):2741–7.
44. Hunt DL, Haynes B, Hanna SE, Smith K. Effects of computer-based clinical decision support systems on physician performance and patient outcomes: a systematic review. J Am Med Assoc. 1998;280(15):1339–46.

45. Evans RS, Pestotnik SL, Classen DC. A computer-assisted management program for antibiotics and other antiinfective agents. N Eng J Med. 1998;338:232–8.
46. Clemens E, Cutler T, et al. Prescriber non-compliance with a new computerised insulin guideline for non critically ill adults. Ann Pharmacother. 2011. http://www.ncbi.nlm.nih.gov/pubmed?term=Clemens%20compliance%20insulin. Accessed in May 2012.
47. Bourgeois FC, Linder J, et al. Impact of a computerized template on antibiotic prescribing for acute respiratory infections in children and adolescents. Clin Pediatr (Phila). 2010;49:976–83.
48. Papaioannou A, Kennedy CC, et al. A team-based approach to warfarin management in long term care: a feasibility study of the MEDeINR electronic decision support system. BMC Geriatr. 2010;10:38.
49. Trafton JA, Martins SB, et al. Designing an automated clinical decision support system to match clinical practice guidelines for opioid therapy for chronic pain. Implement Sci. 2010;5:26.
50. Milner KK, Healy D, et al. State mental health policy: implementation of computerized medication prescribing algorithms in a community mental health system. Psychiatr Serv. 2009;60:1010–2.
51. Tang MB, Tan ES, et al. Electronic e-isotretinoin prescription chart: improving physicians' adherence to isotretinoin prescription guidelines. Australas J Dermatol. 2009;50:107–12.
52. Field TS, Rochon P, et al. Computerized clinical decision support during medication ordering for long-term care residents with renal insufficiency. J Am Med Inform Assoc. 2009;16:480–5.
53. Lesprit P, Duong T, et al. Impact of a computer-generated alert system prompting review of antibiotic use in hospitals. J Antimicrob Chemother. 2009;63:1058–63.
54. Buising KL, Thursky KA, et al. Electronic antibiotic stewardship—reduced consumption of broad-spectrum antibiotics using a computerized antimicrobial approval system in a hospital setting. J Antimicrob Chemother. 2008;62:608–16.
55. Cooley T. Presented at the Guild of Healthcare Pharmacists & UK Clinical Pharmacy Association Joint Conference 2009. Clin Pharm. 2009;1:291.
56. Teich JM, Osheroff JA, Pifer EA, The CDS Expert Review Panel. Clinical Decision Support in Electronic Prescribing: Recommendations and an Action Plan. J Am Med Inform Assoc. 2005;12:365–76.
57. Wang CJ, Marken RS, Meili RC, et al. Functional characteristics of electronic prescribing systems: a field study. J Am Med Inform Assoc. 2005;12:346–56.
58. Miller RA, Gardner RM, Johnson KB, Hripcsak G. Clinical Decision Support and Electronic Prescribing Systems: A Time for Responsible Thought and Action. J Am Med Inform Assoc. 2005;12:403–9.
59. Ammenwerth E, Schnell-Inderst P, et al. The effect of electronic prescribing on medication errors and adverse drug events: a systematic review. J Am Med Inform Assoc. 2008;15:585–600.
60. Summers V. Association of Scottish Chief Pharmacists. Electronic Prescribing – the way forward. Pharm J. 2000;265:834.
61. Trent Rosenbloom S. Approaches to evaluating electronic prescribing. J Am Med Inform Assoc. 2006;13:399–401.
62. Savage I, Cornford T, Klecun E, Barber N, Clifford S, Franklin BD. Medication errors with electronic prescribing (EP): Two views of the same picture. BMC Health Serv Res. 2010;10:135.
63. Green C. Look to the future and see the opportunities. Clin Pharm. 2011;3:34.

Chapter 5
Data Support for Electronic Medicines Management

It is clear from the operational requirements of EP systems that these systems require high quality data inputs from a number of sources. The supporting data for EP systems and other medication management systems fall into four main categories:

1. Patient Data – for example, demographic data such as patient's name, address, date of birth, next of kin, religion etc. These data are usually imported to an EP system from a patient administration system (PAS) and, while patient identifiers, such as name and date of birth are important in the clinical setting, they do not give rise to any design issues specific to EP systems, except possibly at the integration level. For this reason, patient data support will not be considered in any detail in this chapter.

2. Drug Data – for example, medicine name, form, strength, route of administration, synonyms, dose, storage conditions etc. This basic dataset would be required for each prescribed item for a patient. In addition to this indicative information, it is expected that EP systems would provide referential information on prescribed medicines – for example, standard information on contraindications, precautions, side-effects and drug interactions. The accuracy and validation of these data are essential, and issues relating to the implementation of drug data will be discussed at length in this chapter. Some EP systems use their own drug databases, produced in-house from previous implementations; others will use a drug database supplied by a third party data supplier. The source of the drug data has various implications which will be discussed in some detail later in the chapter.

3. Disease and Monitoring Data – for example, diagnostic tools, disease classifications, rating scores and monitoring scales. This type of information is not specifically related to medicines, but it is required in the prescribing process (see Chap. 4, Fig. 4.1), to support disease monitoring, epidemiological reporting and some decision support functions – for example, cancer epidemiology reporting from an oncology system. These data are often readily available in algorithms that are easily codable, but conventions for disease assessment and monitoring can and do change over time, according to guideline, health service and professional body recommendations. It is important therefore that these

S. Goundrey-Smith, *Principles of Electronic Prescribing*, Health Informatics,
DOI 10.1007/978-1-4471-4045-0_5, © Springer-Verlag London 2012

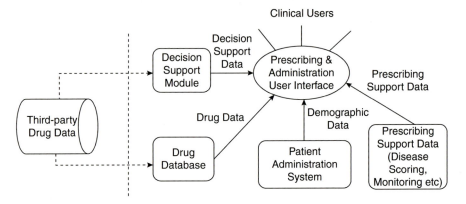

Fig. 5.1 EP system data architecture. The flow of data through an EP system

ancillary data are not hardcoded into an EP system, but are set up as data tables, so that they can be changed when necessary.

4. Decision Support (DS) warnings. As well as the data items described in the first three categories above, which are instantiated in individual patient prescribing records within the EP system, there is a requirement that an EP system provides a system of clinical warnings and alerts for clinical decision support at the point of prescribing. This would include, for example, warnings for drug interactions, sensitivities, duplicate therapies, contraindications and precautions. The warning messages themselves are non patient-specific, in that the same type of message might be used for various different drug interactions for different patients. Consequently, DS functions on EP systems need data tables to store the various clinical alert messages that would be required, and an indexing and querying system to generate the appropriate clinical warnings at the relevant point of the workflow. The data configuration issues relating to DS functions will be discussed in detail later in the chapter. The data architecture of an EP system might be as shown in Fig. 5.1.

In order to gain an appreciation of some of the issues that must be considered in structuring of data support for an EP system, it is helpful for the reader to have a broad understanding of how medicines information reference sources and clinical data coding conventions have developed to the present day. This chapter will examine some of the clinical coding systems and terminologies that have developed, before focusing specifically on the drug data requirements for EP systems, and drug data related issues.

Coding Systems for EP Concepts

As discussed previously, as well as data specifically relating to medicines and their properties, EP systems require data schemas to describe details of diagnosis, contraindications and side-effects, in order to provide the most comprehensive functionality.

The discipline of health <u>informatics</u> has developed to analyse and systematise health and disease related information and, with time, a number of clinical <u>coding systems</u> have evolved to describe health and medicine concepts in a machine-readable manner [1]. Many of the coding systems have their historical origins in the need to classify and enumerate medical events for public health purposes. Many of these have relevance to EP systems and are discussed below.

The <u>International Classification of Diseases (ICD)</u> is a multiple axis disease classification schema which is published and administered by the <u>World Health Organisation</u>. It is now in its 10th revision (ICD 10), but the process is in place for developing the 11th revision [2], which will resolve issues such as usability on web-based systems and integration into electronic health records.

This schema has its origins in the work of William Farr, the first medical statistician for the General Register Office of England and Wales, in the mid-nineteenth century. He saw the need for a classification system for diseases to enable mortality statistics to be collected on an ongoing basis. Initially the schema was designed to record causes of death, but was subsequently developed to list diseases and disorders causing considerable morbidity. The classification continued to be used for the pragmatic purpose of collecting epidemiological data, and is currently used by WHO for making international comparisons of <u>health statistics</u>. The schema is therefore a practical classification, rather than a theoretical one, and it may require adjustments to allow finer levels of detail to be expressed in certain applications. ICD 10 coding is often used as the coding system for diseases and diagnoses assigned to patients in electronic medical records, and would be the point of reference for EP decision support tools giving contraindication/precaution checking or drug-disease interaction checking, based on patient record information. ICD-10 codes are of particular concern in EP applications where there is a clear requirement for production of reports or statistical returns. An example of this would be <u>oncology systems</u> for the management of oncology and haematology clinics, where there is a major political need to report epidemiological data. In the UK, this is facilitated by the agreed <u>National Cancer Data Set</u>, which was established to eliminate reporting inconsistencies between different UK Cancer Registries [3]. The National Cancer Dataset is due to be replaced in 2012 by the Cancer Outcomes and Services Dataset (COSD), which will include the cancer registry dataset, and other site specific data items [4].

<u>Diagnosis Related Groups (DRGs)</u> were developed in the US by the <u>Healthcare Finance Administration</u> as a means of assigning a cost of treatment to a patient's diagnosis. They were developed to enable calculation of Medicaid reimbursement costs. DRGs are based upon <u>ICD Clinical Modification (ICD-CM) codes</u> in ICD 9 or ICD 10. Appropriate ICD codes are refined by placing them in diagnostic categories and then grouping them into subgroups that reflect consumption of resources, criteria for treatment, and potential complications. Thus patients are assigned a DRG from a relatively small number of DRG codes. DRGs are used routinely in the US and have been adapted in other countries where a reimbursement algorithm has been required. They are designed for hospital inpatients and do not provide a suitable means of assessing the costs of <u>chronic disease</u> care. Availability of a DRG designation for a patient, together with actual <u>medicine cost data</u> from an EP system

may permit a variance analysis of projected costs and actual costs of inpatient treatment within the US context.

Read Codes (subsequently called Clinical Terms) were developed in the UK to enable clinicians (mainly in general practice) to code events in the electronic patient record, and thus enable statistical auditing of the patient care process in primary care. Read Codes have latterly been owned and administered by the UK government. Read Codes have changed considerably both in their terminology and in their structure during their lifespan. Version 1 of the Read Codes was a strictly hierarchical schema. In version 2, the structure was changed so that they more closely approximated ICD 9 disease codes and OCPS 4 procedure codes. Version 3 of the Read Codes was, in contrast with v1, a compositional schema, where each term could be augmented by qualifier terms.

Read codes have been used extensively to code for diagnosis, problems and medicine prescribing in GP systems in the UK. However, they have not been used routinely in secondary care applications, largely because they were developed for primary care use. A key issue in the use of Read Codes has been the increasing potential for lack of concept control with combination terms, in the latter versions. However, many primary care (GP) systems map prescribed medicines to their respective Read Codes, and Read Codes may therefore have a role in facilitating communication between primary care and secondary care systems in the UK.

The Systematised Nomenclature of Medicine (SNOMED) is administered by the College of American Pathologists, and was derived from classifications of tumour and pathology nomenclature used by the College. SNOMED is designed to be a comprehensive, computer processable terminology to support all medical concepts. SNOMED is in use in over 40 countries. Principally, it is a hierarchical, multiple axis schema, but it also allows composition of complex terms from simple terms, so is partly compositional, and it has the facility of cross-referencing between terms in the schema. SNOMED International (SNOMED III) incorporates almost all ICD 9 terms, so reports can be generated in ICD 9 format.

In 1999, the College of American Pathologists and the UK National Health Service announced their plan to converge SNOMED and Clinical Terms (Read Codes) v3 into a single terminology. The stated intention was to avoid duplication of effort and to create a universal, international terminology to support electronic patient records. The first version of the combined terminology – SNOMED Clinical Terms – was released in 2002, and was adopted as the standard terminology for UK Connecting for Health healthcare applications [5]. Since 2007, SNOMED CT has been owned by the International Health Terminology Standards Development Organisation (IHTSDO). Third-party drug data suppliers have worked to map their datasets to international terminologies such as SNOMED-CT, in order to provide intraoperability with other systems in the area of more advanced decision support, for example contraindications, dose/indication checking and drug disease interactions.

An important area of data standardisation is the development of HL7 (Health Level 7), which is an XML based terminology [6], designed for the purpose of modelling healthcare processes, and producing a common terminology for all concepts in healthcare, to provide an industry standard for intraoperability across all healthcare applications. Many healthcare IT systems are marketed as "HL7 compliant". However, development of the message formats to enable extensive and comprehensive description of healthcare processes is an ongoing and gradual process. This is because (a) HL7 message formats are being designed to model all healthcare scenarios, not just those involving pharmacy and therapeutics, (b) there is a need for consistency in the consensus-forming process, and (c) major semantic assumptions need to be made and understood by the international HL7 community, at each stage of the HL7 design process in different domains. Recently, there have been initiatives to make closer links between SNOMED-CT concepts and HL7 message formats, in order to achieve greater semantic intraoperability in healthcare applications [7].

Specifically in the area of pharmaceuticals, the Dictionary of Medicines and Devices (dm±d) has been developed to describe concepts associated with the use of specific medicines and devices for the diagnosis and treatment of patients [8]. The dm+d is integrated with SNOMED Clinical Terms and would enable applications dealing with medicines – such as hospital EP systems, and hospital and community pharmacy systems – to exchange information with a common terminology. The dm+d was developed as the medicines terminology for the English Connecting for Health programme. The first part of the dm+d work was the Primary Care Drug Dictionary, which was launched by the UK Prescription Pricing Authority in 2003. The first version of the full dm+d, for medicines used in primary care and secondary care, together with some prescribable devices, was released in 2004. Although the England Connecting for Health programme is being dismantled, dm+d will become the standard for medicines terminology in the UK NHS, and will contribute to the intraoperability of systems in the NHS.

In order to support all aspects of the prescribing, supply and administration of medicines, the dm+d is structured into a number of related concepts, shown in Fig. 5.2.

The dm+d data structure enables EP systems to differentiate at the data level between the concepts of medicine prescribing, administration and supply, which is important to provide rich functionality at each stage in the medicines management process. It will enable users to identify prescribed medicines of the EP system clearly and unambiguously, which will impact on the risk management aspects of EP system use. dm+d will also provide a common platform for analysis of prescribing data in both primary and secondary care in the UK, something that cannot be done at present. This will have important implications for commissioning and care management. Also, comprehensive linkage of dm+d codes with GTIN codes (formerly EAN codes) will enable widespread and reliable use of automation in hospitals and healthcare provider organizations, in conjunction with EP systems.

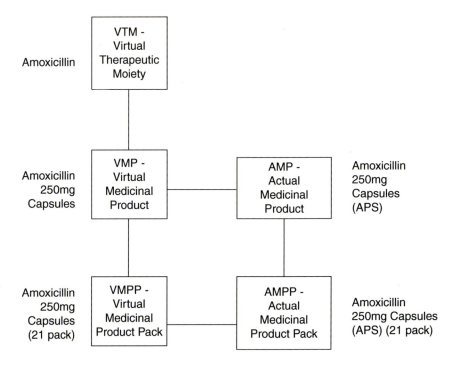

Fig. 5.2 dm+d concept diagram

The Development of Medicines Information Reference Sources

Prior to a discussion of drug data sources for EP systems, it would be beneficial for the non-clinical reader to be aware of the types of medicines information that a prescriber might need to know, and the established reference sources that are available for prescribers and clinical professionals.

Historically, sources of drug information have consisted of

(a) medical and pharmaceutical primary literature from hardcopy journal publications, and
(b) secondary literature, such as recognised pharmaceutical compendia and reference books

The primary literature consists of clinical trial reports, reviews of specific therapeutic issues, case studies and anecdotal reports. The secondary literature consists of drug information compiled from primary sources. This might include recognised reference books, addressing specific clinical issues, such as Stockley's "Drug Interactions", or Briggs' "Drugs In Pregnancy". The secondary literature also comprises of recognised pharmaceutical compendia. A compendium is a book, with a section or monograph, on each listed medicinal product or drug substance. Some of the compendia provide standards for manufacturing and quality control purposes (for example, the British Pharmacopeia and the European Pharmacopeia) and are of little value for prescribers and clinical professionals. Others contain more evaluated clinical information (for example, the Martindale Extra Pharmacopeia), or provide treatment guidelines for rapid reference (for example, the British National Formulary (BNF) or the Monthly Index of Medical Specialities (MIMS)).

Since automated systems have allowed substantial indexed databases to be compiled, stored and retrieved electronically, medical publishers and medical information providers have sought to provide their information sources to end-users in an electronic format. Initially, these electronic products were abstract database services such as the US National Library of Health Medline database, or the Exerpta Medica EMBASE, provided by hosted data services accessed by modem connection – for example, DataStar and Dialog – which enabled remote users to search proprietary databases and information sources. In the last decade or so, with the growth of the internet, many of these database services have become available via web browsers, which have made access far more straight-forward and has simplified searching techniques, enabling a higher degree of end-user access.

Also, with the introduction of optical disk technology over the last 20 years, many of the biomedical databases have been "packaged" and sold as CD-ROM products for single and multiuser use, to enable fast and secure local searching. Many of the pharmaceutical compendia – for example, the British National Formulary or the Martindale Extra Pharmacopeia – are also now available in elec-tronic format, on CD-ROM for single-user or network access.

It should be noted that there are many different databases of medicine-related information that are produced by commercial vendors, professional societies and public bodies, in different countries. An increasing number of these reference sources have been designed specifically for internet use, which enables them to be linked with other systems, and to be accessed by patients and health service end users, rather than health professionals (CKS, Map of Medicine, patient.co.uk). An interesting recent development is the marketing of referential information on medi-cines from a third party data supplier, First Databank Inc, in a web-based browser format for end-user use (FirstLight®).

Examples of some of these are tabulated below (Table 5.1).

In addition to information about medicines produced and compiled by healthcare professional bodies, health providers and the publishing industry, a prime source of information on medicines is from the manufacturers of those medicines. A number of key documents on licensed medicines are produced by the pharmaceutical indus-try and regulatory agencies. These include:

1. The Summary of Product Characteristics (SmPC). This is the definitive docu-ment on a marketed medicine for use by healthcare professionals. It provides a full listing of available data on a medicine in medical terminology.
2. The Patient Information Leaflet (PIL). This is the approved information on a medicine that is available to a patient. The PIL is usually written in plain English,

Table 5.1 Sources of electronic medicines information

Database	Geographical emphasis	Speciality
MedLine	US/UK	Medical research
EMBASE (Excerpta Medica)	Europe	Clinical medicine
TOXBASE	UK	Drug toxicity and side effects
PharmLine	UK	Clinical use of drugs/pharmacy practice research
TICTAC	UK	Medicines identification database
IDIS (Iowa drug information service)	US	Clinical medicine and medicines information
Clinical knowledge summaries (formerly Prodigy)	UK	Treatment guidelines
Map of medicine	UK	Treatment pathways and guidelines
Patient.co.uk	UK	Patient information on medicines

with non technical language. The PIL is included in each medicine pack and, in countries where original pack dispensing is not universal, such as the UK, there is a legal and ethical requirement for the pharmacist to include a copy of the PIL in the dispensed pack.

3. The <u>European Public Assessment Document (EPAD)</u>. This is the document produced by a pharmaceutical company, under the auspices of the European regulatory system, giving a summary of the information supporting the product license application for a medicine.

It is often thought that information provided by the <u>pharmaceutical industry</u> is inferior to that available from independently published sources. However, the required content of the standard medicines documents, the SmPC and the PIL, is now highly controlled and regulated, and therefore these documents form a reliable source of definitive information on a medicine. Furthermore, since the introduction of the structured SmPC format some years ago, much of the information available to health professionals from the pharmaceutical industry in the UK and Europe is presented in a structured way, which could be incorporated into electronic systems. The SmPCs and PILs for UK authorizations are available online in the Electronic Medicines Compendium (EMC).

There is therefore a wealth of information available in various electronic formats concerning the pharmacology and clinical use of medicines. For example, compendial information, such as the British National Formulary or the Physicians' Desk Reference (PDR), is available in internet or CD-ROM form, and therefore links could be made to these reference sources (mounted either on a local network, or on the internet) from an EP system. Indeed, many EP systems have implemented controls to link passively to standard electronic medicines reference sources, in order that these reference sources may be used as explicit decision support tools, although there may be issues concerning licensing in a multiuser situation, or with performance if the reference source is mounted on a remote server. Moreover, <u>medicines information reference sources</u> encoded as XML are particularly suitable for access by EP systems. For example, there is an initiative in the UK to produce PILs in XML format (X-PILs) to enable PILs to be easily adapted to different formats, to enable access by people who are blind or partially sighted [9].

Sources of Drug Databases, and Their Implementation Within EP Systems

However, aside from the licensing and permissions issues involved, many of the available drug data sources that are electronic versions of paper-based references are not used as direct sources of the active drug data that are used in the prescribing workflow of an EP system.

Although electronic versions of hard-copy medicines reference sources constitute high quality sources of medicines data, they are not suitable for use within EP applications for a number of reasons. Firstly, they are compiled for referential purposes, not to support automatic retrieval. This is to say that they are designed for use by a human evaluator and do not have the detailed linkages to support information retrieval by an EP system. Secondly, the data are not structured or defined in an appropriately granular manner for use in an electronic system to support complex prescribing. Thirdly, the data are often not linked with appropriate coding systems to allow interoperability with other systems and to support a variety of advanced functions.

For these reasons, many EP systems use drug databases that are structured to support the functions of the system. The standard data items – drug name, form, strength, synonyms, possible routes, units of prescribing, administration and supply etc. – are all incorporated into data tables within a standard database platform, such as MicroSoft SQL Server. The database tables are structured so as to provide appropriate granularity to permit a range of detailed functionalities (for example, complex prescribing and medicines administration) and are linked in such a way as to provide consistent retrieval of information on medicines and prescribing concepts by the EP system, together with the possibility of incorporating mappings to other drug coding systems (e.g. SNOMED CT, dm+d, Read 2).

The actual drug data used for an EP implementation may be compiled in one of three ways.

(a) The drug database is built for the implementation, by personnel at the hospital site implementing the system. This approach has been taken with certain general clinical systems that have been adapted for the application of prescribing. However, the build process is time-consuming and laborious and it is highly unlikely that the dataset will have the internal consistency of a commercially produced system. Furthermore, the implementing site has the burden of maintaining the system to reflect new products, changes in dose etc. It may be possible to take this approach with an EP or medicines management system with a limited scope of operation, or to support a pilot or prototype study, but it is not feasible for a whole-hospital EP system.

(b) The <u>drug database</u> is adapted from a <u>software vendor's reference database</u>, or a database from another implementation. However, with system providers' in-house databases, there may not be a systematic validation process in place, and the quality of the maintenance process will depend on the expertise and management structures in place within the software provider organisation. Often, with databases built by software houses, where developers may be working both on the software code and the data tables, there may be the temptation to provide some data-related functionality via hard-coded software changes, and thus the boundary between the data and the software can become indistinct. Furthermore, if a database from one EP implementation is used to support a new implementation, it may introduce data that are inappropriate to a different healthcare setting, and errors in the database are perpetuated. Furthermore, if the database has been compiled by a healthcare provider, there may be legal issues surrounding the ownership of the data.

(c) The <u>drug database</u> is structured around, and the data imported from, a <u>third party data supplier</u> dataset. The use of a third party dataset has the advantage that it is more likely to be of a higher quality than a database built by a software vendor or healthcare provider. Third party drug data providers are commercial organisations whose business is to produce databases to support EP systems and other medicines management software, and will have considerable expertise – both clinical and information science – available to them. The dataset of a third party data supplier should be consistent and accurate, with established business processes in place for the compilation and validation of their data. Furthermore, some of these organisations will have external validation, according to quality standards such as <u>ISO 9001</u>. The use of a third party dataset removes the responsibility of maintenance from the EP system vendor, or the healthcare provider (although some data configuration by the software vendor may be required). Also, with a third party data supplier, the legal responsibility for the internal quality of the drug data lies with the data supplier. The major disadvantage with using a third party dataset is the cost of using the data. Typically, a third party data supplier will charge a software vendor for the basic cost of supplying the data, together with an additional charge based on the number and size of sites where the system using the data is in use. These costs are factored into the total contract between the software vendor and healthcare provider, but it still increases the total cost of the implementation. Furthermore, the process of implementing a third-party dataset into a system that has not previously been supported by one will constitute a major technical task, which may deter some EP system providers and their users from migrating to a third party data supplier.

Currently, the most prominent of third party data providers for the provision of drug data to EP and medicine management system suppliers are First Databank Inc and First Databank Europe Ltd, owned by the Hearst Corporation, and Multum, part of the Cerner Corporation. Other sources of drug data include the MicroMedex product range (Thomson Inc), although these products are designed more for use with stand-alone hand-held devices.

Historically, third party data suppliers have not provided referential medicines information to end users, although they have had the capacity to do so; this has been the preserve of the reference sources produced by the publishing sector. However, recently First Databank Europe Ltd has marketed the medicines referential information that supports its decision support functions in a web-based browser format for end-user use (FirstLight®). With increasing data transfer and adaptability, and the need for large information providers to find new markets, this trend is likely to continue.

In the US, some authors have in the past questioned the quality of data from third party data suppliers [10]. However, as commercial organisations whose principal business is supplying medicines data, third party data suppliers review their quality maintenance systems on a continual basis, and are often looking to introduce more advanced functionality. It should be noted too that, in the US, the major centres of excellence for EP systems have the resources and in-house expertise to produce institutional drug databases [10]. However, other smaller healthcare providers do not have the means to produce their own drug reference files and it could be argued that more widespread adoption of EP systems cannot take place without the adoption of third party data sources. Indeed, many of the hospitals in the UK with operational EP systems use data from First Databank Europe Ltd (Exeter) [11, 12].[1]

Requirements of Drug Databases for Supporting EP Systems

The electronic drug dataset forms a key data component of an EP system – this will provide all of the data relating to medicines. In addition to this, other coding and classification systems will be required to support other data elements within an EP system – for example, information relating to indications, contraindications, diagnosis, side effects and monitoring.

However, with EP drug data concepts, there are various potential issues that software designers and implementers should be aware of. Depending on how the EP system database is structured, these issues have the potential to introduce anomalies in the operational use of an EP system. This section reviews some of these issues.

Medicine Nomenclature

Each chemical entity that is used as a medicine ingredient will have an approved name. In the past, all medicines in the UK were routinely named according to their British Approved Name (BAN). However, in 2005, drug nomenclature in the UK was changed to the revised International Nomenclature (rINN) [13]. This change

---

[1] See case studies of Winchester & Eastleigh Hospitals Trust and Shrewsbury and Telford Hospitals Trust in Chap. 2.

Table 5.2 Some examples of British Approved Names (BANs) and their corresponding International Names (rINNs)

Drug type	BAN	rINN
Antibiotic	Amoxycillin	Amoxicillin
Diuretic	Frusemide	Furosemide
Antihistamine	Chlorpheniramine	Chlorphenamine
Anticholinergic (centrally acting)	Benzhexol	Trihexyphenidyl

required <u>third party data suppliers</u> and owners of proprietary databases and medicines information products to change all drug ingredient names from BANs to rINNs on their databases. Common examples of BANs and their corresponding rINNs are shown in Table 5.2.

This change has brought <u>UK</u> medicine nomenclature more into line with that of <u>Europe</u> and the <u>United States</u>. However, the old nomenclature (BANs) still exists in historical records, and there is an argument for retaining the BAN as a synonym (see below) in the database to enable retrieval of historic records. This consideration would also apply to any future specific or general changes of nomenclature.

Designers also need to consider the relationship between a generic name of a product, and the <u>ingredients</u> in the product. Many medicinal products consist of two or more medicine <u>ingredients</u> and, in the UK, many established and most commonly used combination products have an approved <u>combination name</u>. For example, tablets containing a combination of paracetamol 500 mg and codeine 8 mg are called Co-codamol 8/500 tablets. However, many combinations do not have an approved <u>combination name</u>. For example, the antacid combination of sodium alginate 500 mg and potassium bicarbonate 100 mg per 5 ml has the brand name, Gaviscon Advance. In addition, many ingredients of combination products are not available as single entity products; with the above example, sodium alginate is not available in preparations without an acid neutraliser, such as sodium or potassium bicarbonate. There is therefore a need to differentiate the concepts of <u>ingredient</u> and <u>approved name,</u> and to provide the necessary mapping between ingredients and approved name, for each medicinal product. This is important not only for ensuring that medicine descriptors are accurate, but to ensure that the correct decision support warnings for sensitivities, duplicate therapy and drug interactions are flagged for each product.

Synonyms

In drug database terms, a <u>synonym</u> is an alternative name. Regardless of alternative nomenclatures, as discussed above, some drug entities have alternative names that are not branded product names. For example, gonadorelin is also known as gonadotrophin-releasing hormone, GnRH or LH-RH. Given the <u>dm±d</u> hierarchy, it is recognised that brand names of drug entities cannot be regarded as synonyms, since the approved name is a <u>VMP concept</u>, whereas the <u>brand name</u> is an <u>AMP concept</u>. Appropriate synonyms would need to be mapped to each approved name in the database. The use of <u>abbreviations</u> (for example, ISMO for isosorbide mononitrate) is not considered best practice and these should not be listed as synonyms.

Product Mapping

In the UK, general medical practitioners use systems that enable them to prescribe a product by name at the <u>AMP concept</u> level. Thus the prescription generated states "Amoxicillin 250 mg/5 ml SF Liquid – 100 ml – One 5 ml spoonful three times a day". It is clear to the pharmacist exactly what product needs to be supplied against the prescription and, indeed, with the UK system, this is necessary so that the pharmacist can claim the appropriate reimbursement for dispensing the product.

However, hospital doctors usually prescribe at the <u>VTM concept</u> level. A hospital prescriber would write "Amoxicillin 250 mg po (by mouth) three times a day", and would not specify the actual product in many cases. Hospital EP systems therefore face the challenge of translating the prescriber's VTM prescription to an AMP dispensed item. This process is achieved through two mechanisms within an EP system:

(a) By the mapping of VTM, VMP and AMP terms within the EP system database
(b) By structuring the <u>prescribing workflow</u> of the EP system so that it forces the prescriber to be as specific as possible with the details of the order. This has to be balanced against the number of steps in the workflow that the prescriber has to complete.

Pharmaceutical Forms

In primary care, a relatively small number of pharmaceutical forms are used – for the most part, these are: tablets, capsules, inhalers, oral liquids, creams, ointments and lotions. Secondary care prescribing, however, includes a wider range of forms – for example, implant, bone cement, or impregnated stent. It is important that all possible pharmaceutical forms are included in an EP system database, using standard nomenclature. However, care must be taken that route of administration concepts are not combined with form concepts within the data – for example, "subcutaneous injection". Also, proprietary terms for certain pharmaceutical forms – for example, "Respule®", should be avoided, in favour of a generic concept (in this example, "inhalation capsule"). Consideration should also be given to how two different forms of the same medicine, supplied in the same pack would be expressed by the system – for example, Canesten Combi, an antifungal product that contains a clotrimazole pessary and a clotrimazole cream.

Routes of Administration

As with pharmaceutical form, a much wider variety of routes of administration are used in secondary care than in primary care, and it is important that all the routes of administration that are likely to be used are reflected in the database. The EP system must be able to support the following route-related scenarios:

(a) administration of the same product by different routes, either concurrently or sequentially.
(b) administration of the same product by alternative routes – for example: metoclopramide 10 mg injection, to be given intramuscularly *or* subcutaneously.

Dose Information

Consideration should be given to the way in which doses are expressed within EP systems. While the standard SI unit for a drug dose is milligrams, and the abbreviation "mg" is used, the recommendation is that drug doses are expressed as mg as far as possible and that, where other SI units are used, they are not abbreviated. Examples of this would be: (a) Digoxin 125 µg tablets, (b) Alfacalcidol 250 ng capsules.

EP systems need to differentiate between <u>dose units</u>, <u>administration units</u> and <u>supply units</u>. In order to operate a medicines administration module, an EP system needs to map the dose expression to the administration expression. Thus, for Flucloxacillin 500 mg capsules, a dose of "1 g three times a day" would translate to an administration instruction of "two capsules three times a day". The supply units are important if there is a direct feed to a pharmacy system, and supplies are being made automatically. Unit doses such as tablets and capsules can also be supplied in the quantities that they are administered in, and this will enable electronic unit dose dispensing in countries where it is the norm. However, for many products, the supply unit cannot be directly equated to the dose and administration unit. For example, in order to fill a prescription for "Salbutamol 100 µg Inhaler – two puffs to be inhaled four times a day", the smallest unit that can be supplied is a 200 dose inhaler. Also, antibiotic liquids would be supplied in quantities of 100 ml, because they have to be reconstituted and, because of their shelf life, it is not practical to use them for another patient's supply, in the same way as some other liquids. In any case, many topical products – for example, such as creams and ointments, consist of a definite supply quantity (100 g tube), but with <u>indeterminate dose and administration quantities</u> (one application), so that the number of dose/administration aliquots making up the supply quantity cannot be calculated.

In order for dose information to be transmitted between systems, to facilitate intraoperability, there is a need for standard <u>dose syntax</u>, where information on doses is transmitted as an agreed format/concatenation rather than as free text. Work is ongoing to develop a <u>dose syntax model</u> for the UK NHS, in conjunction with HL7, to resolve this intraoperability issue [14].

Admixtures

As well as medicines that are fixed dose combination products throughout their product life, consideration should be given to those products that are essentially mixtures, originating from two separate products. In some cases, where the two individual products are mixed together at the point of <u>medicines administration</u> (for example, an intravenous admixture, such as the commonly used mixture of the antibiotics, cefuroxime and metronidazole), it is probably best for the two products to remain listed as separate entities at the database level, and for the EP system to have functionality to combine more than one medicine on the same order, so that the prescriber can specify the mixture, as opposed to the individual products, at the point of prescribing. In other cases, where the product is supplied as a mixture of two active agents (for example, <u>extemporaneous products</u> such as Coal Tar in Betnovate 0.1% Ointment) it is better to list the mixture as a product in its own right on the database. This is especially the case if one of the ingredients is not routinely administered therapeutically to the patient as a separate product (Coal Tar Solution BP in the above extemporaneous example).

Some admixtures will have two or more variable ingredients. An example of this would be <u>Total Parenteral Nutrition (TPN)</u> – intravenous feeding solutions. These will have a nitrogen/protein component, a carbohydrate/energy component and a number of vitamins and minerals as trace elements, and the constituents would vary according to the patient's clinical and nutritional requirements. Sometimes a finite number of fixed regimens will be used – especially if a hospital routinely buys in TPN regimens from commercial providers, and in this case, the specific fixed combination regimens could be listed as single entities on the database. However, if there is continuous variability with TPN requirements, it would be appropriate to have the fluid and trace element formulations listed separately in the database, and to have TPN compounding functionality within the EP software for the pharmacy user to formulate custom regimens. However, TPN functionality represents an advanced functional area in EP systems.

Non-indexed Products

While there are a wide variety of medicines, pharmaceutical forms and routes of administration used in hospital prescribing that are not used in community prescribing, there are also a large number of products usually prescribed and supplied by pharmacies in primary care, that might not be prescribed, and supplied by pharmacy, in hospitals. These would include items such as non-medicated dressings, colostomy products and dietary products. In some healthcare contexts, it may be appropriate for these non-acute products to be included on a hospital EP system for accounting purposes. Nevertheless, in other situations, they may be considered out of scope of the hospital EP system.

However, all of these products would be included in an update from a third party data supplier. There is therefore a need to designate a proportion of a data update as "non-indexed". This may be done either by (a) assigning non-indexed products to some sort of dump file, away from the main database structure, or (b) by leaving them in the main data structure, but rendering them invisible to the end user. The former method may lead to retrieval problems if a non-indexed product needs to be retrieved from the dump file and placed within the active database. The latter method provides a consistent data structure but, depending on other factors, the performance of the drug database may be affected by large numbers of invisible records.

Third party datasets resolve many of the structure and consistency issues described here, according to their established rules, and through mapping to the various terminologies that are in use. For example, First Databank Europe's MDDF Product Set groups the relevant products (AMP concept) for each generic (VMP concept) term, within its dataset. So, for "Atenolol 50 mg tablets", the Product Set would include all of the Atenolol 50 mg tablet presentations from different manufacturers.

Many of the terminology-related issues here are subject to ongoing standardisation initiatives at European and international level – for example, ISO TC 215. Nevertheless, these standardisation initiatives often involve a considerable number of stakeholders, and a balloting process, and so they are necessarily slow, and not optimally responsive to new developments or drastic changes in professional practice. Furthermore, the process of standard development is often dominated by system vendors, who have a vested interest to ensure that the standard is closest to the functionality provided by their own system. Standards are often, therefore, compromises and may embody ambiguities which will find their way into EP systems datasets [15].

Data for Decision Support Tools

As well as the drug database, third party data suppliers will often provide data and messaging for clinical decision support (DS) functions. Typically, these will include sensitivities, drug interactions, drug-disease interactions, duplicate therapy warnings and precautions. When a medicine is prescribed for a patient, the EP system will query the other patient- and medicine-related data, and return any clinical warnings about the prescribing of that medicine, in relation to other medicines prescribed and other patient factors.

Take, for example, a system for sensitivity or allergy checking. Using an EP system, a patient is prescribed the antibiotic, amoxicillin, for a chest infection. However, it has been recorded in the patient's electronic record that they are allergic to penicillin, and amoxicillin belongs to the penicillin group of antibiotics. In order to perform an allergy check, the EP system needs to run a query, or use a query tool or decision support engine, which registers the allergy information in the patient data, and the drug name, which is associated with the drug data, and gives a warning message to the user, as a result of this match.

In order to support DS functions, the structuring of the DS ruleset and the indexing of drug and patient data should be done in such a way as to ensure consistent retrieval. Using the above example, if a patient is allergic to penicillin, then the system should also show an allergy warning if pivmecillinam is prescribed, even though it is slightly different in structure to other penicillin antibiotics. Again, using the above example, the system should consistently recognise known cross-sensitivities. Therefore, if a patient is allergic to penicillin, then an appropriate warning should flag up if the patient is prescribed a cefalosporin antibiotic, for which there is a 10–20% probability of cross reactivity with penicillins.

The accuracy and reliability of clinical alerts is a key consideration in the implementation of DS tools. In the past, various implementers have chosen not to introduce any DS functions in their EP system at all, rather than set up a DS system that does not have an adequate data platform or appropriate granularity in the data.[2]

Another issue is that many DS tools on proprietary systems may display large numbers of warnings that may be of questionable clinical significance. A common example of this is the display of reciprocal warnings with drug interactions (the user is warned that there is an interaction between aspirin and warfarin, and also between warfarin and aspirin). The risk issues associated with warning fatigue are discussed at length in the previous chapter. However, the display of excessive warnings may be an indicator that the indexing methodology is not sufficiently refined, and improving the indexing methodology may well rationalise the querying process, and thus improve the performance of the system.

While accuracy of clinical warnings, and appropriate inclusion of warnings in the prescribing workflow is a key consideration for risk management and implementation of best practice within the organisation, research has shown that the end user is primarily concerned with speed of response, i.e. the performance of the system [16]. Implementers need to consider how DS data is structured within an EP system database and transmission of queries between different parts of the system, as these factors affect the speed of operation.

Some implementers have attempted to build basic decision support functions from first principles within EP applications, in particular those applications that are designed for general order communications, rather than medicine prescribing and administration specifically. This approach, however, is very laborious, in the same way as building a custom drug database. Furthermore, the resulting DS system is unlikely to be comprehensive or fully consistent in its operation. On the other hand, implementation of a third-party DS system into an EP system may be a difficult task from a technical perspective. For this reason, some third party data suppliers provide the DS ruleset as a "toolkit" which serves as a "black box" so that developers do not have to produce complex querying routines to support the DS functions. All they need to do is route the queries into the toolkit, and a DS warning response will emerge from the toolkit for display at the front end.

---

[2] For example, the implementers at Southmead Hospital, Bristol (see paper by Gray S., Smith J), and at the Winchester & Eastleigh NHS Trust, prior to the adoption of a third party dataset.

Legal Issues with EP Data

It is an important principle in systems analysis that the function of the software and the accuracy and integrity of the data handled by the software cannot be considered in isolation. This is certainly the case with clinical systems, which seek to facilitate the patient care process by automation, because the correct outcome is dependent on both the software and the data, and errors made by the system could cause harm to the patient. With an EP system, it is of no value to have a well-constructed workflow for the prescribing and administration of medicines, if the drug data used to formulate the prescriptions generated are full of errors and inconsistencies.

As mentioned previously, there are essentially two approaches to setting up a drug database to support an EP/medicines management application – to build a database specifically for the application, or to implement a third party drug database. There are legal implications, however, with both of these approaches. If a drug database is built for a specific application by a software vendor, then the software supplier is the legal owner of the data and they structure, implement and deploy the data as they wish. However, there is a requirement for the software vendor to maintain that database, and ensure that it is fit for purpose on an ongoing basis. The software supplier is legally liable for any clinical errors arising from use of the software when the data are inadequate. For this reason, the supplier should have robust procedures for the maintenance of the clinical data, and should have clinically-qualified personnel involved in the processing of the data. Some software vendors use a reference dataset that has been built by one particular healthcare provider, as the basis for further implementations. As mentioned previously, this can cause problems due to perpetuation of errors, and use of a dataset designed for one organisation within another organisation. From a legal perspective, the originating healthcare provider is the legal owner of the dataset, even if the software vendor is subcontracted to maintain the site databases, which could lead to difficulties in the event of a dispute between the healthcare provider and the software vendor.

On the other hand, third party data suppliers bear legal responsibility for drug data that they provide, as long as the data are implemented within client systems according to their recommended specifications.

Conclusion

Availability of high quality data – relating to the patient, the medicines and the prescribing process – is essential for the correct operation of EP software. A variety of formal coding and classification schemes exist to manage the data that may be required in EP systems. There are numerous sources of medicines information data, but only some of these are available electronically and structured in a suitable way to support EP applications. Furthermore, issues arise with the way such data are implemented within an EP system. Many systems use a drug data source from a third party data supplier to resolve some of these issues. A major issue in data support for EP systems is the development of common data standards and conventions, as this is the key to interoperability of these systems.

References

1. Coiera E. Guide to health informatics. 2nd ed. London: Arnold; 2003. p. 202–22.
2. Ustun TB. Presented at Australian Health & Welfare Institute Meeting, Towards ICD 11 for Australia, University of Sydney. 2011. http://www.aihw.gov.au/TwoColumnWideLeft. aspx?pageid=10737419473
3. Pheby DF, Etherington DJ. Improving the comparability of cancer registry treatment data and proposals for a new national minimum dataset. J Public Health Med. 1994;16:331–40.
4. National Cancer Intelligence Network. Cancer outcomes and services dataset. 2011. http:// www.ncin.org.uk/collecting_and_using_data/data_collection/ncds.aspx. Accessed in November 2011.
5. NHS Connecting for Health. Electronic prescribing in hospitals: challenges & lessons learnt. 2009. p. 74. http://www.connectingforhealth.nhs.uk/systemsandservices/eprescribing. Accessed in November 2011.
6. Kabachinski J. What is health level 7? Biomed Instrum Technol. 2006;40:375–9.
7. Ryan A, Eklund P, et al. Toward the intraoperability of HL7v3 and SNOMED CT: a case study modelling mobile clinical treatment. Med Info. 2007;12:626–30.
8. Frosdick P, Dalton C. What is the dm + d and what will it mean for you and pharmacy practice? Pharm J. 2004;273:199–200.
9. Voss J. Launch of the X-factor for the visually impaired: the X-PIL. PIPA J. 2006;5:4–6.
10. Miller RA. Clinical decision support and electronic prescribing systems: a time for responsible thought and action. J Am Inform Assoc. 2005;12:403–9.
11. Barker A, Kay J. Electronic prescribing improves patient safety – an audit. Hosp Pharm. 2007;14:225.
12. Gray S, Smith J. Practice report – electronic prescribing in Bristol. Healthc Pharm. August 2004:20–2.
13. Anon. Changes of drug names from BANs to rINNs. Pharm J. 2002;272:364.
14. Anon. Dose syntax. 2011. http://www.dmd.nhs.uk/dossyntax.html. Accessed in November 2011.
15. Hammond WE. The role of standards in electronic prescribing. Health Aff (Millwood). 2004;Web exclusive:W4-325-7.
16. Bates DW, et al. Ten commandments for effective clinical decision support: making the practice of evidence-based medicine a reality. J Am Med Inform Assoc. 2003;10:523–30.

Chapter 6
Electronic Medicines Management: Support for Professional Practice

The changing role of the various professions in the health services provides implementers of EP systems with the challenge of how professional roles are recognized and regulated within an EP system. This will be discussed further in Chap. 7, concerning the use of EP systems by non-medical prescribers. However, if systems are to be accepted by users, designers and implementers will also need to consider how EP systems will support, or can be configured to support, the needs of healthcare professionals in their everyday practice.

Modernization of Healthcare Working Practices

As mentioned in Chap. 1, EP systems have the potential to revolutionize the working lives of healthcare professionals by facilitating changes in working practices. Because EP systems enable routine processing and dissemination of prescription information in an automated way then, depending on software design and hardware availability, systems can be used to support new and different ways of working.

Of the healthcare professionals that are principal stakeholders in the implementation of electronic prescribing, medical and nursing staff have traditionally had the most contact with patients in hospitals. On the contrary, pharmacists have in the past been departmentally based, at a distance from patients, since historically their role has revolved around the dispensing and supply of medicines.

However, over the last 30 years, there has been a paradigm shift in hospital pharmacy practice. This has been especially the case in the UK, but the same trend has been present in other countries. There has been a decline in the importance of the manufacturing and formulation aspects of the hospital pharmacist's role, and a corresponding increase in the significance of the pharmacist as an advisor in medicine use, working closely with patients and staff at ward level, to ensure the safe and effective use of medicines.

S. Goundrey-Smith, *Principles of Electronic Prescribing*, Health Informatics,
DOI 10.1007/978-1-4471-4045-0_6, © Springer-Verlag London 2012

This paradigm shift in pharmacy practice has been stimulated by a number of factors:

(a) The increasing complexity (and cost) of new therapeutic advances, and the range of therapeutic interventions available, necessitating an increased reliance on clinical evidence in therapeutic practice. These changes in clinical pharmacology have been supported by the growth of the medicines (drug) information services over the last 30 years, and the adoption of <u>electronic medicines reference sources</u> by these services.

(b) The increasing expectations of patients concerning information about the benefits and risks of their treatment, together with the availability of information on medicines from other sources (e.g. the internet). These changes have increased the significance of the pharmacist as an expert on medicines, providing high-quality medicines information. Moreover, patient expectations have been positively encouraged in recent years, with a greater emphasis on consumer choice and effective healthcare driven by the notion of the "<u>empowered patient</u>", and also the <u>personalization</u> of medical care, where care plans are made personal to individual needs.

(c) The loss of so-called <u>Crown Immunity</u> in UK NHS hospitals in the early 1990s. From this time onwards, hospitals were no longer exempt from the <u>Medicines Act 1968</u> legislation governing the manufacturing activities of the <u>pharmaceutical industry</u> and so, instead of controlling their own manufacturing activities, hospital pharmacy based manufacturing units were required to obtain a manufacturer's license and be subject to regulatory inspections in exactly the same way as the pharmaceutical industry. This has curtailed manufacturing activities in UK hospitals.

The emphasis on <u>near-patient clinical activities</u> has increased in recent years for US hospital pharmacists too, and many forms of innovative clinical pharmacy activity are documented in the American hospital pharmacy literature.

The nursing profession also has undergone a paradigm shift, from being traditionally a labor-intensive vocational occupation, subservient to medicine, to being a degree-educated profession, with an increasing amount of clinical autonomy, and political significance. In many countries, nurses have recognized clinical specialties, manage specific clinic services, are active in health promotion and <u>health education</u>, and have prescribing responsibilities (the specific implications of which will be discussed further in the following chapter). With these new roles, nurses have gained a new political significance in many health economies, not least in the UK NHS, where the nursing professional bodies have been at the forefront of promoting new roles and responsibilities for nurses, and the nursing profession has had an increasing impact on the provision of routine healthcare and <u>health screening</u>, and provision of health education to the public.

Hospital <u>doctors</u> have faced a number of challenges in recent years, which have had profound implications for their professional practice. Firstly, the armamentarium of diagnostic and therapeutic techniques available to specialist clinicians is steadily expanding, both in terms of cost and technological complexity. There is therefore a need for physicians to keep up to date with new technologies and new procedures. Secondly, while there is an increasing number of effective medical interventions, in many countries, in particular the UK and Australia, there is a shortage of doctors. This is exacerbated by the political pressures to reduce the contracted working hours of doctors, for reasons of patient safety, and changes to medical career planning. As a result of this, there is increasing willingness within health provider organizations to delegate routine tasks that have traditionally performed by junior doctors, to other healthcare professionals. While there is good rationale for this, in terms of appropriate use of "skill mix", some physicians feel that patient care is compromised, and that their professional identity is threatened. Moreover, some studies have suggested that the continuing professional development needs of those health professionals engaged in providing new services have not been fully understood and addressed.[1]

EP Systems: Support for Professional Practice

It is clear that, in twenty-first century healthcare systems, health professionals are facing various professional and political challenges, and that professional roles are changing. Nevertheless, healthcare professionals are still committed to providing optimum patient care, according to best standards of practice, and in the light of an adequate evidence base. On this basis, there is a clear potential for electronic prescribing system to support and enhance clinical practice, both in terms of optimizing current practice, and supporting and developing new roles and services. A number of papers have discussed the capacity of EP systems to support and enhance professional practice, within the health professions.

Pharmacy-led evaluations of EP systems have recognized the potential of EP systems to support ward-based clinical pharmacy activities and interventions. Marriott et al. [2] undertook a study in the UK comparing the number and type of pharmacist interventions at Queens Hospital, Burton on Trent (BH), where a fully integrated patient data and prescribing management system has been implemented, as discussed previously [3], and Good Hope Hospital, Sutton Coldfield (GHH), where a traditional paper-based system was in place. Over a period of 2 months in 2003, a larger number of clinical interventions were made at BH – 2,512 interventions (equivalent to 0.2 interventions per finished consultant episode (FCE)), compared to 763 interventions (0.05 interventions per FCE) at GHH. Furthermore, the types of intervention were different between the two hospitals. Thirteen percent of the pharmacist interventions at GHH, the paper-based hospital were concerning drug interactions, use of non-formulary medicines, route changes and prescription legibility, but there were no interventions of this type at BH, the hospital with the EP system,. However, at BH, 26% of interventions were concerning medicines information and patient monitoring, whereas there were no interventions of this type at GHH.

---

[1] For example, with nurse prescribers. See Courtenay et al. [1].

Because the workload and case-mix of the two hospitals was similar, as was the patient demographic profile, the authors concluded that the EP system facilitated more clinical pharmacy interventions. Considering also the different profile of interventions between the two hospitals, there may be three factors involved:

(a) The EP system, with its decision support tools, automates the prescribing process, and therefore eliminates errors associated with choice of drug, prescription legibility etc.
(b) Because various types of intervention relating to the actual prescribing and supply procedure are reduced, pharmacists have more working time available to devote to near-patient clinical activities – monitoring new treatments, assessing side effects, and providing advice to other healthcare professionals – which will in turn give rise to other types of intervention.
(c) The EP system presents a larger amount of clinical data in a systematic manner and therefore facilitates the identification of hitherto unrecognized intervention issues by clinical pharmacists.

Traditionally, data on pharmacist interventions has been collected to justify the existence of clinical pharmacy services. However, clinical pharmacy services are now well established and there is a need to take the evidence-base a step further to see how clinical pharmacy interventions actually affect patient outcomes. However, this requires a robust data-capture procedure, and paper-based monitoring systems have usually been too laborious and haphazard to provide a validated and benchmarked dataset on pharmacist interventions. A project has been conducted in five NHS Hospital Trusts in Wales, UK [4] where a personal digital assistant (PDA) database has been used to report pharmacist interventions. Pharmacists across the Trusts entered intervention data over a 2 week pilot period, resulting in the collection of data on 1,531 interventions, from 38 hospital wards. The PDA clinical intervention system was a quick and convenient way to collect intervention data. Furthermore, the dataset was useful for identifying inconsistencies between different Trusts at the enterprise level, and comparing the practice of pharmacists in different clinical specialties. An EP system would provide the potential for the clinical intervention record, logging interventions by all professionals, to be held alongside, and integrated with, the prescribing record.

The introduction of tools to specifically support the work of clinical pharmacists is an important aspect of EP system design, and only pharmacists can drive forward the availability of such tools in EP systems [5]. American hospital pharmacists have long recognized the potential of electronic prescribing and computerized decision support systems to support clinical practice in pharmacy. In her discussion on the potential for computerized physician order entry (CPOE) to enhance pharmacy practice, Shane [6] indicated that, in 2002, a number of health providers in the US had already implemented centralized and decentralized automation to increase the efficiency of the prescribing process and medicine supply process, and therefore enable pharmacists to concentrate more on pharmaceutical care. Indeed, since financial pressures faced by health providers would focus managers' attentions on pharmacist headcount once CPOE was implemented, there was a pressing need for the pharmacist's role to be redefined.

Shane [6] indicated that US health system pharmacists had traditionally focused their attentions on medication management during acute disease -during a patient's hospital stay – and that lack of time and information had precluded any attempt to manage a patient's chronic disease medication requirements on a long-term basis. However, EP systems can now make chronic disease management possible, and this will have implications for the role of the pharmacist, and the pharmacist's required professional competencies, and therefore continuing professional development needs.

This requirement represents a particular economic burden in the US, where there are large and disparate ethnic groups of people with chronic diseases, many of whom are not receptive to health education messages, are poor, and are reliant on State medical insurance (Medicaid/Medicare). Nevertheless, those with chronic diseases undoubtedly represent an equally significant challenge to the health economies of the UK, continental Europe and Australia. EP systems have the potential to address issues relating to chronic care, and change the professional practice of healthcare professionals accordingly.

As discussed previously, the nursing profession has undergone significant changes, and nurses have taken on new roles and responsibilities. While it has been recognized that nurses are a key stakeholder in the implementation of an EP system,[2] [7] and their attitudes to the introduction of an EP system can be influential in its acceptance, there is little documentation on the role of electronic systems in helping nurses develop their professional roles.

Nevertheless, EP systems can benefit nurses in their routine duties. The introduction of the closed-loop process electronic prescribing system at a London Hospital [8], where medicines administration working practices were revised following the introduction of barcode patient identification and automated ward dispensing cabinets ("magic cupboards"), caused the medicine administration round time to be decreased from 50 to 40 min. There was a corresponding increase in nursing time spent on medication related issues outside of drug administration rounds, but this might reflect appropriate redeployment of skills as a result of automation. A systematic review of the impact of electronic health records on time spent on documentation by nurses and physicians [9], it was found that the use of bedside terminals and desktop PCs at the nurses' station reduced nurse documentation time by 24.5% and 23.5% respectively, during the course of a shift. However, this decrease in nursing time was offset by a considerable increase in physician time per shift, when physicians used desktop PCs for CPOE.

The main area of interface for nursing staff with an EP system is the medicines administration functionality. It is important, therefore, that this part of the EP system is designed to be as user-friendly as possible for nursing staff doing their drug

---

[2] The attitudes of nursing staff were noted as being a key factor in the adoption of the Winchester EP system (see Case Study in Chap. 2).

administration round on a busy ward. A key element of this is that the medicines administration screen looked as much like a traditional drug chart as possible.[3] Another important element is that the medicines administration screen is designed in such a way that all of the drug administration instructions and annotations are clear, unambiguous and easy to read.

Nurse specialists will have involvement in activities such as clinic management, medicines review and clinical audit; all of these could be facilitated by specialist advanced functionality within EP systems. These are discussed in detail in later sections of this chapter. The role that EP systems can play to help support nurses in supplementary and independent prescribing roles is discussed fully in the next chapter.

The potential impact on EP systems on physician practice has been extensively discussed in the literature. Many of the benefits of electronic systems to physicians concern the use of decision support systems to assist with the prescribing process, and the ability of CPOE systems to reduce medication errors within hospitals [10, 11]. Both of these benefits should reduce the likelihood of a doctor facing litigation as a result of a medication error, and automate the routine processes of therapeutics, in order that clinicians can concentrate on the intuitive, human aspects of medicine. EP systems have also been shown to reduce financial costs and hospital stay time [12, 13] which would be a benefit to clinicians with responsibility for budget management in their clinical area. Furthermore, as already noted, there is emerging evidence that EP systems may be having some impact on patient outcomes in chronic diseases, due to their effects on routine clinical practice [14]. However, as noted previously, it is likely that these organizational benefits are specific to the healthcare context in which they were elucidated.

Nevertheless, not all changes facilitated by EP systems are positive. Some studies point to the way in which CPOE increases physician prescribing time [9, 12] due to the design of the prescribing workflow. Also, it has been noted that decision support systems may not always be effective because they do not fit appropriately into the prescribing workflow, or do not flag up latent physician monitoring needs [15].

Nevertheless, the electronic capture of the prescribing history by an EP system, together with the possibility of interfaces between the EP system and other systems and devices opens up a range of potential applications that might benefit medical practice. These might include automated data downloading for clinical audit and management reporting, remote clinics and the use of hand-held devices for domiciliary visits, clinical trial data collection and prescribing support.

It has been suggested that EP systems can change the dynamics of a patient's consultation with a prescriber (doctor or other healthcare professional) [16]. Historically, the prescriber has "led" the consultation, imparting information to the patient, who has been in a passive role. With a comprehensive EP system, where the

---

[3] This was found to be a key user requirement at Winchester. Also, at Burton on Trent, the fact that system screens looked like forms that staff were already familiar with was an important factor in the acceptance of the system.

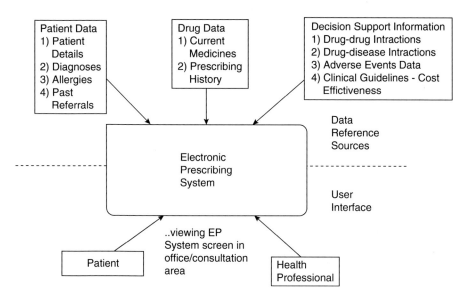

Fig. 6.1 A new dynamic. Patients and healthcare professionals can be partners in the prescribing and medicines management process using the EP system, as they view the medicines information together (See Schiff and Rucker [16])

system can be used to retrieve medicines information, as well as prescribe the medicine, however, there is the potential for the prescriber and the patient to view the same screen (so called "triadic consulting") [17]. The prescriber can therefore talk the patient through the benefits and risks of the medicine to be prescribed, and the rationale for prescribing, using medicines information material retrieved from the EP system, or hospital intranet, while at the same time setting up the prescription for the patient. This is illustrated in Fig. 6.1.

The remainder of this chapter will discuss some of the specific ways in which electronic prescribing systems support clinical professional activities.

Audit Logs in EP Systems

The audit logs within an electronic system represent a major tool for data gathering to support professional practice, and manage operational issues in a health within a healthcare provider organization. Three published studies of UK EP implementations have highlighted the usefulness of the audit trail that an EP system can provide [18–20]. The underlying audit functions of an EP application keep a log of all operations performed on the software, with a record of the operator, date and time of each operation. Thus, for any prescription, the user and time details are stored relating to initial creation of the prescription, subsequent amendments to the prescription, acknowledgement of clinical warnings, doses administered, and other significant points in the life of the prescription. Here, the term "audit" is used in a specific IT-related context, as opposed to clinical audit, a separate issue which will be discussed in detail in the next section.

Audit logs are a useful feature of an EP system as they may be used to

(a) investigate critical incidents relating to errors in prescribing and medicines administration, and to identify "near miss" situations, where a change of procedure would be beneficial.
(b) provide management information on the prescribing process and to resolve specific disputes concerning supply and administration of medicines.
(c) provide information on EP system user behavior, which may be beneficial for future developments and enhancements of the system, as well as for guiding planners of user training and professional development.

They may even be useful in providing evidence of malpractice; at the Wirral hospitals [18], a nurse was arrested for unauthorized prescribing using a doctor's log-in details, because the doctor could prove he was not present at the hospital at the time the unauthorized prescribing took place, as evidenced by the system audit log.

A key consideration with audit trails in EP is that the database is designed with appropriate audit logging tables in it at the outset, in order to provide a sufficiently comprehensive dataset to support audit trails, and the extent to which the audit logging and reporting functions can be configured to each hospital site.

Use of EP Systems for Clinical Audit

Over the last 20 years, medicine has become increasingly an evidence-based activity and now software applications are able to collect information on clinical activities within a hospital in an increasingly efficient manner. It is now relatively straightforward for a manager or clinician to obtain management reports of procedures undertaken or medicines administered in a hospital, with numbers and details of each event. These reports are used as the basis for clinical audit, whereby clinicians and managers review the information concerning a drug or procedure, to determine the activity level and cost of the intervention, and an estimation of whether the intervention is being done in accordance with local or national clinical guidelines, or accepted best practice for the profession concerned.

In many health environments, there are financial pressures limiting allocation of health resources, and practitioners are under pressure to justify their professional practice, in the eyes of patients and other stakeholders, and also to demonstrate that their interventions have an objective benefit to patient care. Thus, for many healthcare professionals, clinical audit is a useful tool, and has profound political significance.

Traditionally, the data for clinical audits have been obtained by a variety of means. For analysis of hospital admissions, a specific report would be generated from the patient administration system (PAS), based on a search for the coded data entity for the diagnosis or admission type from the patient records. For a review of surgery performed within a hospital, an electronic health record would be queried on the basis of the OPCS procedure codes associated with each patient record. For some very specific audits of clinical services, data have been collected manually using questionnaire or observational techniques.

Audits of medicine use generally seek to answer questions that managers and clinicians might have about cost-effective and appropriate use of medicines, across the whole population of patients who are admitted to hospital. Audits may be conducted to evaluate the following scenarios:

(a) For a relatively expensive medicine, an audit of drug use could address the following questions:

- how many dose units are being used, and of which formulation? (tablet or injection)
- where the drug is being used, is it being used according to the manufacturer's recommended dosage schedule, or in line with any existing clinical guidelines within the hospital?

The results of such an audit may be used to establish a guideline for use of the drug in the hospital, if such a guideline is not already in existence.

(b) The extent to which patients commenced on intravenous antibiotics are transferred to equivalent oral antibiotics after 2 days of intravenous dosing. The transfer to oral antibiotics after a short IV course is recommended in order to minimize treatment costs, to prevent the emergence of resistant pathogens and reduce the risks associated with intravenous therapy. A clinical audit of the route of antibiotic administration would monitor compliance to local clinical guidelines, identify exceptional cases and determine whether there are any consistent features of exceptional cases that could be remedied.

To conduct audits of medicines use, there have, in the past, been two basic approaches. Firstly, a standard starting point has been a product/formulation use report from the pharmacy system, as this would provide a reasonably accurate picture of medicines being issued from the pharmacy, and would be relatively easy to obtain from a pharmacy system. Such reports could be used as the basis of product use comparisons between different wards and specialties. However, the number of packs or dose units issued by the pharmacy, as evidenced by reports from the pharmacy computer system, does not necessarily correspond to actual administration of dose units to patients. Discrepancies may be caused by:

(a) the use of when required (prn) medicines, such as analgesics and antiemetics, where the consumption by the patient is variable and where there may be little correlation to the number of dose units issued by the pharmacy.

(b) The use of <u>ward stock</u>. A stock supply to a ward, issued by pharmacy, might be used on a variety of patients, depending on the ward's pattern of admissions.

(c) The administration of a single dose of a medicine to a patient, as an emergency measure, where the medicine given was borrowed from another ward or department outside of pharmacy opening hours, and therefore would not be reflected in the pharmacy issues to that ward. This issue would also occur with the use of <u>patient's own drugs (PODs)</u> within the hospital, a practice that is common in the UK, as a means of reducing <u>hospital expenditure</u> on patient's long-term medicines which are unlikely to be changed during the course of an acute admission.

In order to surmount the problem of the relationship between doses issued by the pharmacy and actually administered to the patient, a second approach to clinical audit is therefore for ward-based staff to record the number of actual dose units of a medicine administered to a patient. This approach has the advantage that it would gather an accurate record of all medicine doses administered to a patient – be they when required (prn), single doses, or from stock packs. However, with the traditional system of using paper <u>drug charts</u> for recording administration of medicines, the record of all dose units administered would need to be transcribed manually to audit documentation. By this method, recording administration events for all patients on a ward just for one drug formulation would be a laborious process. Such a manual recording process is far too labor-intensive to produce the variety of ad hoc reports of medicine use that may be needed in a routine operational environment.

In addition, there are specific problems arising from the <u>manual transcription</u> or rekeying of medicines administration data from paper drug charts:

(a) Due to the legibility of charts, it may not be clear what dose was administered and on what date.

(b) If details of administration are being recorded in the audit, the prescriber's administration instructions on the chart may be sufficiently ambiguous that it is not clear how exactly the medicine has been administered on each occasion.

(c) If a prescriber has specified multiple routes for a medicine (e.g. metoclopramide 10 mg im/pr/po prn) in a single prescription, it may not be clear from the administration record which route was used for which administration event.

(d) When manually transcribing administration events, inconsistencies in the data may be introduced due to assumptions made by different transcribers.

EP systems with full medicines administration functionality offer the possibility of comprehensive querying functions for conducting clinical audits. Such a system is able to capture data on dose units administered to a patient, at the point of administration, thus providing a detailed an accurate record of medicine consumption for a ward, specialty or subgroup of patients.

Furthermore, if an EP system is interfaced with the <u>pharmacy system</u>, it is theoretically possible to reconcile the stock issued from the pharmacy with the doses actually administered to patients, and to analyze the variance. An accurate usage review will be harder to perform for items that are not issued for a specific patient (stock items). However, usage reviews for drugs issued to specific patients would be helpful for monitoring wastage of mid-price, mid-volume items, and for analyzing patterns of use of prn drugs.

There are, however, a number of issues that may affect the ability of an EP system to facilitate comprehensive clinical audits/drug use reviews:

1. There may be problems with mapping data on products issued by the pharmacy with records of doses administered at ward level. This may be due to inconsistencies in pack sizes for the same product, or anomalies in PIP codes or GTIN codes assigned. This may also be because the pharmacy system and the EP system may have different ways of handling the drug data.
2. There will be a proportion of prescriptions where the administration instructions will be in a free text format, because they are more descriptive. These prescriptions cannot be retrieved in the same way as prescriptions with coded administration instructions in an audit process.
3. It has been observed with some EP systems [18] that once only (stat) medicines may be administered in an emergency situation, but may not be subsequently recorded on the system. This may lead to an artificially low record of drug use in an audit.
4. Consideration would need to be given to the practicalities of extracting and collating drug usage data for audit purposes. Reporting software, such as Crystal reports, is useful for extracting data from an application database, in order to facilitate flexible reporting, but a certain level of IT competence is necessary to set up the reports required. Furthermore, there may be issues with collating the data if a report is compiled from two physically distinct databases – for example, the EP system database and the pharmacy system database. If the data elements are compatible, it may be possible to import the required data from the two databases into temporary tables, so that the reporting software can query the combined dataset. Alternatively, the reporting tool would need to be run against each separate database and the reconciliation of data from the two sources performed further down the process.

While many healthcare systems have used Crystal reports in the past, there are now a number of newer reporting applications that have been introduced specifically for medicines management, such as ReportPLUS and HPAS [21].

EP Systems and Patient-Centered Medicines Reviews

As well as clinical audit and drug use review, which seek to answer questions about the general use of medicines across a population, for management and budgetary purposes, an area that is of increasing interest to many healthcare professionals is the performance of patient-focused, structured medicine reviews. With such a review, the patient is interviewed by the healthcare professional, so that the healthcare professional can obtain a prescribing history for that patient and can identify any issues relating to side-effects or compliance. The reviewer then may make recommendations to the prescriber concerning possible dose adjustments or discontinuation of medicines.

Questions that a structured medicines review may seek to answer are as follows:

(a) Whether a prescribed medicine is appropriately indicated for a patient.
(b) Whether medicines are being prescribed at the correct dose and frequency for the indication.
(c) Whether there are significant side effects with any medicine.
(d) Whether there are any significant drug interactions or drug sensitivities that may be giving rise to side effects.
(e) Whether what is referred to as "polypharmacy" (the accumulation of therapy due to inappropriate overuse of drugs or inappropriate treatment of side effects) can be reduced.

Structured medicines reviews have grown in their importance during recent years, and their significance is subject to some controversy. While it has been claimed that medicines reviews can improve health outcomes, some studies have failed to demonstrate the cost-effectiveness of pharmacist-performed medicine reviews [22].

The role of the medicine review came to the fore in the UK NHS following the publication of the UK government National Service Framework for the Elderly [23] in 2001, which recommended that every patient over 70 years of age on four or more regular medicines should receive a medication review every 6 months. Hospital pharmacists have traditionally provided feedback to prescribers about appropriate use of medicines in a reactive manner; however, in the UK, comprehensive medicines reviews in hospitals, in a proactive manner, are still not being carried out consistently across a range of specialties and geographical locations [24].

Since EP systems will have a clear and accurate record of the medicines prescribed for a patient, together with proactive and reactive decision support tools, EP systems have the potential to support healthcare professionals in conducting patient-centered, structured medicines reviews.

An EP system might have medicine review functionality as part of the pharmacy workflow, or alternatively, as a separate module within the application. The outline functional flow for medicines reviews might be as follows:

(a) The reviewer selects the patient record for review. There is a facility for the patient's consent to the review to be recorded.
(b) The system will then display the profile of currently prescribed medicines for that patient.
(c) The system would then guide the reviewer through a structured review process. For each prescribed medicine on the profile, the system would advise the reviewer of any significant clinical checks (drug interactions, drug disease interactions, sensitivities, duplicate therapies), and would direct the reviewer to any appropriate care plans or clinical guidelines for treatment. The likely scenario is that these decision support tools used in the medicines review process would be driven from the same decision support database used by the EP system for proactive decision support at the point of prescribing.

(d) For each medicine, the system would also prompt the reviewer to ask the patient relevant questions for each medication. Responses from the patient would then be entered into the system.

(e) The information from the review would then populate a predefined medicine review form, which may be a healthcare provider standard format document. The system would prompt the reviewer with suggested recommendations to the prescriber, either to be included on the medicine review form as they stand, or to be overridden by the reviewer on the basis of their clinical experience.

(f) The completed medicine review form would then be routed to the prescriber and would be displayed for action by the prescriber when the patient's record is next accessed.

It is anticipated that the medicine use review functionality would be operated by the reviewer on a wireless laptop PC, tablet PC or palm PC, so that they can conduct the review interview with the patient at their bedside on the ward, or in an outpatient clinic situation. As with medicine administration functions, a personal digital assistant (PDA) would not be adequate for this application due to the small screen size.

One of the problems noted in the use of medicine reviews so far, especially in the community situation, is the effective communication of medicine review information from reviewers (usually pharmacists) to prescribers. One of the advantages of an EP system facilitated medicines review process in hospitals is that it is possible for the review process to be designed and implemented in consultation with, and taking into account the needs of, both prescribers and reviewers. In this way, the process will be acceptable and relevant to all stakeholders, and is more likely to be used effectively. Furthermore, the recommendations of the medicines review are available directly to the prescriber in electronic form, linked to the relevant patient record, which may increase the likelihood of the review being acted upon. Future, more sophisticated systems might offer functionality to link medicine review recommendations to prescribing routines. Then, if the prescriber accepts the recommendations of a review, by clicking on the relevant parts of the review form, new or amended prescriptions are automatically generated, which are then authorized by the prescriber.

An EP system can therefore facilitate a closed loop process for medicines review, whereby a review is initiated with an accurate prescribing history for a patient, and conducted in a structured and consistent manner, with inputs from the system's decision support tools. Specific and well-defined recommendations are then made to the prescriber and, if the prescriber chooses to accept the reviewer's recommendations, the recommendations are then implemented by the EP system in an accurate and consistent manner. The process can then be repeated with future reviews in an manner (Fig. 6.2).

It is clear that, due to the use of decision support tools at the point of prescribing, electronic prescribing will lead to more rational prescribing at the outset [11], which will obviate some of the issues that present in medicines reviews at the current time. However, the extent to which electronic prescribing affects subsequent medicine reviews has not yet been fully elucidated. In any case, there is an important role for healthcare professionals in conducting patient-centered medicine reviews, in order to identify ongoing issues with side-effects, compliance and other aspects of

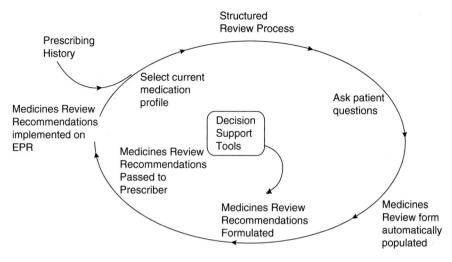

Fig. 6.2 Closed loop medicines review process

pharmaceutical care (e.g. inhaler technique). The "closed loop" review process, which can be supported by an EP system, will support health professionals as they develop this part of their professional practice and may improve patient outcomes relating to these reviews, which will help to resolve controversy relating to the efficacy of medicine reviews.

Involvement of EP Systems in Clinical Research

Clinical research is an important aspect of medicine use in hospitals, and an important element in the professional development of healthcare professionals. This is true for all healthcare professionals, but especially the case for the medical profession. In order to advance within a specialty, or to gain a higher degree (e.g. MD), doctors are required to undertake some clinical research in their specialist field.

Because of their ability to capture clinical data at the point of care, EP systems have the potential to be of value to health professionals involved with therapeutics-related clinical research.

The EP system could be used to perform the following tasks:

(a) Identification of a cohort of patients being treated with a particular therapeutic intervention (either an individual medicine, a particular dose of an individual medicine, or a recognized regimen of several agents). The demographics of the patient and the duration of the therapeutic intervention may also be taken into account.

(b) Generate the necessary documentation for an ethics committee submission, and maintain a record of ethics committee approval.

(c) Flag up patients fitting the trial criteria to the investigator as potential clinical trial patients, or alternatively flag up patients who would not be suitable for enrolment, due to the trial exclusion criteria.

(d) Maintain a consent record for each patient in the cohort, and an ethics committee approval record for the cohort.

(e) Flag up a warning to other prescribers accessing the patient's record in the EP system that the patient is enrolled in a clinical trial.

(f) Assign trial medication to each patient, with a "sealed envelope" de-blinding function, if it becomes necessary to identify whether the patient is taking active or placebo medication.

(g) Provide decision support to prescribers concerning concomitant medication prescribing [25], or other clinical trial violations, in order to prevent attrition of patient numbers in the trial, which is a common problem in some specialties [26].

The patient data could then be exported to a database or clinical trial management application for subsequent processing. Alternatively the data could be maintained within the EP system, as part of a specific clinical trial module. Once the patient data is in a database designed for the clinical trial, either within the EP system or elsewhere, observational data could then be downloaded for each patient from PDAs used by healthcare staff attending the patient. It has been demonstrated that handheld devices, such as PDAs, are an effective and accurate means of gathering observational data for clinical trial patients at the point of care [27].

A few studies have looked at the benefit of IT support in the management of clinical trials. Formea et al. [28] has described how electronic medication order sets can enhance the care of patients in clinical trials, as they can eliminate hard copy documents which cannot be fitted into hospital processes, and provide electronic protocol-specific templates which incorporate local prescribing requirements and an agreed review and approval process. Seroussi and Bouaud [29] have described the use of the Oncodoc system, a browsing tool using a decision tree knowledge base, which matched patient details to available clinical trial protocols. The system was found to be successful in improving protocol compliance, and increasing patient involvement in clinical trials.

EP systems therefore have the potential to screen potential candidates for therapeutic clinical trials effectively and accurately, thus improving the quality of the trial database, streamlining the data collection process, and increasing the viability of the trial as a whole, and the likelihood of a meaningful outcome.

EP Systems: Support for Continuing Professional Development

All healthcare professionals have a duty of care to their patients, in law, and therefore have an ethical responsibility to provide patient care according to the most current clinical evidence, and in line with accepted best practice for their profession.

In all developed countries, there is increasing emphasis on the professional regulation of healthcare professionals, together with an awareness of a greater risk of litigation if negligence can be demonstrated. For these reasons, continuing professional development (CPD), where health professionals are required to keep abreast of the latest clinical and professional developments in their profession, has assumed greater significance for the health professions. The CPD process should be firmly rooted in the realities of practice and many adult educationalists will advocate the use of a reflective cycle type approach [30], which enables the practitioner to take an aspect of their current practice, learn something from it, and bring that learning to bear on future practice. Some health professionals are required to undertake a specific number of hours of CPD, or a certain number of "CPD events" per year. In some cases, completion of a structured CPD record is a prerequisite for professional reaccreditation, so that the health professional can continue in professional practice.

An EP system will contain a wealth of healthcare practice-related information – patient prescribing histories, care pathways and clinical guidelines, decision support information and disease monitoring information. Consequently, such systems have the potential to support CPD for healthcare professionals in a variety of ways, which might include a specific CPD module for clinical multiple choice questionnaires (MCQ), an integral CPD record, or links to professional body CPD websites, and use of the system to provide case histories or simulations.

A key consideration in the design of CPD support functions for an EP system is that CPD events should arise from practice and that the learning gained from the CPD is then reapplied to practice. It is important therefore that there is a facility for CPD functionality to be launched from any screen on the EP system that a healthcare professional is working from, in a way that does not impede their workflow.

The potential role of the EP system in the training of non-medical prescribers will be discussed at length in the next chapter. However, EP systems are able to facilitate the development of prescribing skills and knowledge in all professional groups involved with medicine prescribing.

Integrated Care Pathways and Clinical Guidelines

As discussed, EP systems have the potential to apply specific clinical guidelines or care pathways automatically to the prescribing process, as part of the decision support (DS) tools (see previous chapters). Because of the increasing emphasis on evidence-based medicine in clinical practice, together with the growing need to allocate resources and to regulate costs of treatment, government agencies see EP systems as a means of mandating the use of clinical guidelines and appropriate regimens for different medicines.

However, research on DS tools has shown that clinicians will not adhere to clinical guidelines, even when those guidelines are good, unless the guidelines are integral to a <u>prescribing workflow</u>, in a useable manner [31]. That is to say, the system has to be structured in such a way that the prescriber has to view and act upon the guidelines before they can prescribe medicines. As discussed in earlier chapters, there is a balance between implementing a <u>workflow</u> that forces the prescriber to produce an accurate prescription, and one that has too many steps to be workable in a busy clinical environment. However, if care pathways and guidelines can be successfully integrated into the <u>prescribing workflow</u> in an EP system then, not only are they likely to be followed, they are likely to be memorized and to have an impact on professional practice.

Another issue is the use of <u>web-based hospital formularies</u>, which are usually mounted on a hospital intranet site. There is the potential to link an EP system with the intranet-based hospital formulary. Furthermore, this could be done in an advanced manner so that, when the therapeutic options in a particular care pathway are selected, a list of formulary-approved medicines is preferentially available to be prescribed. This would mean that supplementary prescribers and less experienced independent prescribers are guided by the EP system in an evidence-based manner.

EP Systems: A Gateway to Medicines Information Reference Sources

As discussed in Chap. 5, published sources of drug information have in the past consisted of the medical and pharmaceutical primary literature from hardcopy journal publications, together with secondary reference publications, such as recognized compendia – for example, the <u>Martindale Extra Pharmacopeia (Martindale)</u>, and <u>Stockley"s Drug Interactions</u> – and periodicals – for example, the <u>British National Formulary (BNF)</u>, or the <u>Monthly Index of Medical Specialties (MIMS)</u>. Now, however, many of the <u>pharmaceutical compendia</u> – for example, the BNF or Martindale – are available in electronic format, on CD-ROM for single-user or network access.

There are also many medicines reference tools that are web-based, such as the Map of Medicine or Clinical Knowledge Summaries, which could be linked in to EP workflows.

While, as previously discussed, these reference sources are not generally useful for supporting the drug data requirements of the EP system itself, they are well-respected sources of detailed, impartial medical information for health professionals, and have an important role in supporting clinical practice for all professionals who are involved with the prescribing and supply of drugs.

These resources will have a beneficial effect on professional support and development if they are available in electronic form to the health professional within the clinical system in a way that facilitates easy access. EP systems with ward-based clinical workstations make this a possibility.

Conclusion

All healthcare professionals conduct their professional activities within recognized legal and ethical constraints. Furthermore, it is recognized that healthcare professionals should seek to follow what is accepted best practice for their profession, as determined by peer evaluation. These are the marks of a profession. However, for many clinical professionals, the professional role is changing, due to changes both in society and within healthcare provider organizations. EP systems have the potential to facilitate best practice for clinical users and to be the framework for new professional roles and service provision.

References

1. Courtenay M, Carey N, Burke J. Independent extended and supplementary nurse prescribing practice in the UK: a national questionnaire survey. Int J Nurs Stud. 2007;44:1093–101.
2. Marriott J, Curtis C, et al. The influence of electronic prescribing on pharmacist clinical intervention reporting. Int J Pharm Pract. 2004;12(Suppl):R44.
3. Curtis C, Ford NG. Paperless electronic prescribing in a district general hospital. Pharm J. 1997;259:734–5.
4. Adcock H. Electronic solution to intervention monitoring aids clinical governance. Hosp Pharm. 2006;13:137.
5. Goundrey-Smith SJ. Electronic prescribing – technology designed for the healthcare setting. Pharm J. 2007;278:677–8, 683.
6. Shane R. Computerized physician order entry: challenges and opportunities. Am J Health Syst Pharm. 2002;59:286–8.
7. Willson W, Buisson J. New IT demands new ways of working. Pharm J. 2003;272:33.
8. Franklin BD, O'Grady K, et al. The impact of a closed-loop electronic prescribing and administration system on prescribing errors, administration errors and staff time: a before and after study. Qual Saf Health Care. 2007;16:279–84.
9. Poissant L, et al. The impact of electronic health records on time efficiency of physicians and nurses: a systematic review. J Am Med Inform Assoc. 2005;12:505–16.
10. Bates DW, Gawande AA. Improving safety with information technology. N Engl J Med. 2003;348:2526–34.
11. Hunt DL. Effects of computer-based clinical decision support systems on physician performance and patient outcomes. J Am Med Assoc. 1998;280:1339–46.
12. Tierney WM, Miller ME, et al. Physician inpatient order writing on microcomputer workstations: effects on resource utilisation. J Am Med Assoc. 1993;269:379–83.
13. Evans RS, Pestotnik SL, et al. A computer assisted management program for antibiotics and other antiinfective agents. N Eng J Med. 1998;338:232–8.
14. Michelis KC, Hassouna B, et al. Effect of electronic prescription on attainment of cholesterol goals. Clin Cardiol. 2011;34:254–60.
15. Bates DW, et al. Ten commandments for effective clinical decision support: making the practice of evidence-based medicine a reality. J Am Med Inform Assoc. 2003;10:523–30.
16. Schiff GD, Rucker TD. Computerised prescribing: building the electronic infrastructure for better medication usage. J Am Med Assoc. 1998;279:1024–9.
17. The Good Practice Guidelines for GP Electronic Patient Records. Department of Health, Royal College of General Practitioners, British Medical Association. 2011, v4, p. 174. http://www.

connectingforhealth.nhs.uk/systemsandservices/infogov/links/gpelec2011.pdf. Accessed in November 2011.

18. Farrar K. Accountability, prescribing and hospital pharmacy in an electronic, automated age. Pharm J. 1999;263:496–501.

19. Gray S, Smith J. Practice report – electronic prescribing in Bristol. Healthc Pharm. August 2004:20–2.

20. Foot R, Taylor L. Electronic prescribing and patient records – getting the balance right. Pharm J. 2005;274:210–2.

21. Richman C. How to get useful information out of drug reports – and save time. Clin Pharm. 2011;3:186–8.

22. Pacini M, Smith RD, et al. Home-based medication review in older people: is it cost-effective? Pharmacoeconomics. 2007;25:171–80.

23. National Service Framework (NSF) for Older People. London: Department of Health; 2001. http://www.dh.gov.uk/en/Publicationsandstatistics/Publications/PublicationsPolicyAndGuidance/DH_4003066. Accessed in May 2012.

24. Slee A, Farrar K, Hughes D, et al. Electronic prescribing – implications for hospital pharmacy. Hosp Pharm. 2007;14:217–20.

25. Dale M, Goundrey-Smith S, Higham S, Collinson A. Reducing human error in checking concomitant medications. J Clin Res Best Pract. 2010;6:1–5.

26. Collin C, Davies P, Mutiboko IK, Ratcliffe S. Randomised controlled trial of cannabis-based medicine in spasticity caused by multiple sclerosis. Eur J Neurol. 2007;14(3):290–6.

27. Fischer S, Stewart T, et al. Handheld computing in medicine. J Am Med Inform Assoc. 2003;10:139–49.

28. Formea CM, Picha AF, et al. Enhancing participant safety through electronically generated medication order sets in a clinical research environment: a medical informatics initiative. Clin Transl Sci. 2010;3:312–5.

29. Seroussi B, Bouaud J. Using oncodoc as a computer-based eligibility screening system to improve accrual onto breast cancer clinical trials. Artif Intell Med. 2003;29:153–67.

30. Morris K, Safdar A, et al. Make reflection part of your daily practice. Clin Pharm. 2010;2:397.

31. Bates DW, Kuperman GJ, Wang S, et al. Ten commandments for effective clinical decision support: making the practice of evidence-based medicine a reality. J Am Med Inform Assoc. 2003;10:523–30.

Chapter 7
Electronic Medicines Management and Non-medical Prescribing

Background to Non-medical Prescribing

Traditionally, in healthcare, the prescribing of medicines has been the preserve of the doctor. In the UK, the right to prescribe medicines was assumed by the medical profession following the 1858 Medicine Act and, during the century that followed, the roles of the health professions in relation to medicines have become well demarcated: doctors prescribed medicines, pharmacists dispensed or supplied medicines and nurses administered medicines. This distinction has persisted across the health professions, especially in secondary care, until relatively recently.

However, over the last 20 years, prescribing by other healthcare professions has been developed in a number of countries – the United States, Canada, Sweden, Australia and New Zealand, as well as the United Kingdom [1]. A number of social and economic factors have contributed to the development of non-medical prescribing:

(a) government concerns in various countries about shortages of doctors;
(b) the need to expand channels of prescribing in order to meet public health targets in certain disease areas;
(c) the need to make the best use of the "skill mix" among the professions of the NHS, given their respective numbers and manpower issues, and
(d) a decline in the paternalism with which the public regard the medical profession, together with the political empowerment of other healthcare professions.

The remainder of this section will describe the development of non-medical prescribing, and the issues it entails, specifically in the UK context. Space does not permit full discussion of the development of non-medical prescribing in other healthcare economies.

As discussed, doctors have traditionally been the prescribers of medicines, and, in the UK, the Medicines Act, 1968, limited the legal right to prescribe medicines to doctors, dentists and veterinary surgeons. However, in 1986, the UK Government's

S. Goundrey-Smith, *Principles of Electronic Prescribing*, Health Informatics,   137
DOI 10.1007/978-1-4471-4045-0_7, © Springer-Verlag London 2012

Table 7.1 Prescriber types and user roles

Professional group	User role	Prescriber type	Formulary prescribing permissions
Doctor	Consultant – renal medicine	Independent prescriber	Renal medicine specialist formulary
Doctor	Foundation stage (F1/F2) doctor – surgery	Independent prescriber	None
Pharmacist	Purchasing pharmacist	Non-prescriber	None
Pharmacist	Clinical pharmacist – surgery	Supplementary prescriber	None
Pharmacist	Consultant pharmacist – asthma care	Independent prescriber	Respiratory medicine specialist formulary
Nurse	Clinical nurse specialist – oncology	Independent prescriber	Oncology & hematology specialist formulary
Nurse	Staff nurse – surgical ward	Non-prescriber	None

This table shows a brief schema for designation of hospital EP system users. A schema with this level of granularity may be used to support specialist formulary prescribing as well as non-medical prescribing

Cumberledge Report – "Neighbourhood Nursing – A Focus for Care" identified the potential of non-medical prescribing. This report advocated prescribing by community nurses within their sphere of competence, and led to the establishment of the Advisory Group on Nurse Prescribing in the UK, chaired by Dr June Crown. This group conducted two reviews of prescribing (known as "the Crown Reports"), which have been key to non-medical prescribing in the UK. The first Crown Report recommended that nurses with a district nurse or health visitor qualification should be able to prescribe from a limited formulary, and also that nurses should be able to supply medicines within "group protocols" (i.e. where a group of patients who fulfill certain criteria can be given a certain type of medicine on written instructions from a doctor or dentist). The second Crown Report defined the two key types of prescribers – *dependent* prescribers, or supplementary prescribers, and *independent* prescribers (see Table 7.1).

Dependent, or supplementary, prescribing – prescribing to a patient-specific clinical management plan (CMP) set up by an independent prescriber – was introduced for nurses and pharmacists in 2003. This was the extended to chiropodists/podiatrists, physiotherapists, radiographers and optometrists in 2005.

The first form of nurse independent prescribing was prescribing by community nurses from the Nurse Prescribers Formulary (NPF), which was piloted in 1994 and rolled out in 1998. The second form of nurse independent prescribing allowed nurses and midwives with additional prescribing training to prescribe from an extended formulary, a development which took place in 2002. From 2006, all extended formulary nurse prescribers have become nurse independent prescribers and can prescribe from a full formulary (within their area of competence and if authorized by their employer).

The first pharmacist independent prescribers began their training in 2006. Pharmacist independent prescribers can prescribe from a full formulary, with the exception of controlled drugs.

Experience of Non-medical Prescribing

There is now considerable documented experience with the work of non-medical prescribers. In 2004, a review of 18 papers was published describing the impact of the first phase of nurse prescribing, using the Nurse Prescriber's Formulary (NPF) [2]. The consensus of this review was that patients were generally satisfied with nurse prescribers, and that the nurse prescribers were happy with their role, albeit with some concerns about their pharmacological knowledge. However, the review highlighted prescribing variations between the types of nurse prescriber at that time (district nurses, practice nurses and health visitors) and the limitations of the NPF.

There are also published reports of specific clinics that are led by non-medical independent prescribers, primarily nurses and pharmacists. These clinics tend to be in well-defined specialties and are led by non-medical prescribers who have developed clinical expertise in that field and who generally work with a limited range of medicines.

Some examples of clinics led by non-medical independent prescribers that have been reported in the literature are sexual health clinics, diabetes clinics and asthma clinics run by primary care nurses and diabetes clinics and rheumatology clinics run by specialist hospital pharmacists [3, 4].

In these clinics, non-medical prescribers will take professional responsibility for all prescribing decisions, together with review of a patient's condition, and case-load management. Furthermore, there is a clear framework of referral for patients who encounter specific complications and who might need a medical referral, or the attention of a more experienced clinician.

Benefits and Risks of Non-medical Prescribing

There are a number of clear benefits of non-medical prescribing. Firstly, clinics led by non-medical prescribers are an important means by which services from health providers can be expanded, at a time when resources are subject to an increasingly limited budget. Secondly, these clinics can facilitate an appropriate redistribution of the work load, in order to best utilize the various skills of health provider staff (the "skill mix" issue). Thirdly, a review of nurse extended formulary prescribing in 2005 [5] indicated that, in general, patients were satisfied with nurse prescribing. Many patients valued the way that non-medical prescribing improved access to treatment, although half of the patients said that they would still prefer to see a doctor for certain conditions. As part of the review, an expert panel examined a sample of observed consultations. The panel found that the nurse prescribers observed were prescribing medicines in a clinically appropriate way and were adequately communicating information to patients about the medicines, and exploring the patients' beliefs about treatment. This might reflect a perception on the part of patients that non-medical prescribers might have more time to spend with each patient than doctors.

Notwithstanding the various benefits of non-medical prescribing, in terms of appropriate use of skill-mix, expansion of healthcare services, and improved access to treatment, a number of areas of risk have been highlighted with non-medical prescribing. These concerns center on safety and clinical governance issues:

Patient Safety

The patient safety aspects of prescribing by non-medical prescribers have been extensively discussed over the last 20 years as nurse and pharmacist prescribing has been rolled out. However, the fact remains that there are few comparative data on the rates of prescribing errors with prescribers of different professional groups. Moreover, it is recognized that there is a percentage of avoidable errors with medical prescribing. A recent study commissioned by the UK General Medical Council [6] showed that the prevalence of prescribing errors made by hospital doctors was between 7% and 10%. All grades of doctor (including consultants) made some prescribing errors but unsurprisingly, the highest rate of prescribing errors was among the foundation grades.

As discussed previously, it is recognized that electronic prescribing and electronic health records reduce medication errors, including prescribing errors [7, 8]. It is envisaged then that this benefit could be realized for all types of prescriber, using an integrated prescribing workstation in an EP system. This would certainly be the case if there were specific tools in the EP system to support and manage workflow for particular types of non-medical prescriber.

However, while supportive of non-medical prescribing in general terms, the Committee on Safety of Medicines has expressed some concerns about non-medical prescribing, around the area of records access and management [9]. The first issue was whether all prescribing professionals would have full access to the patient's records prior to prescribing, something that is a key prerequisite to making a clinically appropriate prescribing decision. The concern was that, while surgery, health centre or hospital based staff would have access to patient records, peripatetic healthcare professionals and those who are community-based would not. Following on from this, if an EP system was in use, then certain non-hospital-based prescribers would subsequently not be able to log their prescriptions onto the system, if they did not have remote access. The second issue is concerning how access to prescribing records would be coordinated where there are multiple prescribers who may be working on a patient record. These logistical concerns may be addressed by the system architecture and logic of an EP system.

Training of Non-medical Prescribers

Concerns have been raised about the training of nurse and pharmacist prescribers in areas that have traditionally been the preserve of medicine, for example history taking, assessment and diagnostic skills. Given that some of the concerns about training of non-medical prescribers are because independent and supplementary prescribing courses are too short in duration, the training of non-medical prescribers has implications for undergraduate education, as well as postgraduate education, in those disciplines. However, it should be remembered that, equally, there are potential training issues for medically-qualified prescribers. Traditionally, pharmacology and therapeutics has been taught to medical students as a factual discipline, but the recent trend in medical education has been towards problem-based learning and away from the factual approach. There is therefore the potential for medical education in pharmacology and therapeutics to reflect more closely the realities of clinical practice, and for there to be some integration of therapeutics training for all major health professionals – i.e. a core syllabus at basic/undergraduate level. This opens up the possibility of the use of an EP system to facilitate prescribing and therapeutics training.

The potential for EP systems to support training and continuing professional development (CPD) was discussed at length in the previous chapter. Nevertheless, there are certain ways that EP systems can assist with the training needs of non-medical prescribers – for example, use of care plans, incorporation of clinical guidelines, access to medicines information reference sources, and simulation training.

Clinical Governance

From an organizational perspective, healthcare providers need to have a robust system of clinical governance in place for the regulation of all prescribing activities, including the management and facilitation of non-medical prescriber led services. These would include the following:

(a) information on the scope of competence and responsibility for different non-medical prescribers
(b) records of the training, CPD and professional accreditation and professional insurance details of named non-medical prescribers
(c) clinic procedures, with audit and risk assessments and, in particular, a procedure for management of critical incidents.

The advantage of an EP system is that many of these governance requirements can be embedded in EP functionality in a seamless way, so that the software will support non-medical prescribers, without giving the negative impression that it is restrictive to their activities.

Role of EP Systems in the Management and Support of Non-medical Prescriber-Led Services

As discussed in previous chapters, electronic prescribing systems have the potential to automate routine aspects of prescribing workflow, and to revolutionize working practices. There is now some evidence looking at the benefits and risks of electronic prescribing implementations from the perspective of different professional groups using the system. McVeigh [10] found that an EP system is beneficial for optometry prescribing both to prevent medication errors and adverse drug events, and also to encourage compliance with care regimens and guidelines and good administration/claims management for the health provider. With the Birmingham University Hospitals EP implementation, Slee [11] noted the potential of the EP system to facilitate compliance with local policies and guidelines, for example a hospital antibiotics policy.

Consequently, many EP systems have the potential to address some of the above risk management issues associated with non-medical prescribing, and thus have a role in supporting and enhancing the practice on non-medical professionals who are involved in prescribing.

However, there is evidence to suggest that different professional groups use an EP system in different ways. Niazkhani et al. [12] interviewed physicians, pharmacists and nurses in a Dutch hospital and found that the EP system fragmented medicines-related information and created a number of issues around integration of professional workflows, which caused professional groups to bypass the system in some scenarios. They concluded that all professional workflows needed to be fully integrated with the core physician workflow. Therefore, as with other benefits of EP systems, the capacity of a system to support different prescriber workflows adequately is critically dependent on system design. The design areas that would need to be considered are described below.

EP Systems and Role-Based Access (RBAC)

An electronic prescribing system will usually have a comprehensive function set for managing user permissions and logons. As discussed in previous chapters, this is essential, not only for the security of the system and the data on it (which is sensitive personal information), but also to control access to functionality and to generate an audit trail of user activity, which can be used to create management reports and to track critical incidents.

The granularity of the user permissions management function set is critical in the design of functionality to support different prescriber types. In a typical EP system, each user will have a role assigned to them, which is often based on their professional group – e.g. doctor, pharmacist, nurse. These general groupings may then be subdivided into more specific groups, as shown in Table 7.1.

However, in order to support prescribing by professional groups other than doctors, the user permissions management dataset will also need to map prescriber type against each professional group. Thus, for each user name, there would be fields for (a) profession (e.g. pharmacist), (b) role (e.g. clinical pharmacist) and (c) prescriber type (e.g. independent prescriber).

Thus, for a user with the user profile of pharmacist/clinical pharmacist/independent prescriber, the system would allow access to EP functionality at three levels – (a) for pharmacists – e.g. verify/clinical check, pharmaceutical care planning;

(b) for clinical pharmacists – e.g. management of <u>specialty formularies</u>, drug use review/<u>clinical audit</u> functions, and (c) for pharmacist independent prescribers – e.g. prescribing rights, probably from a specialist formulary, after input of <u>professional accreditation</u> and <u>training</u> details for that user. Consideration should be given to possible <u>role conflicts</u> that might occur in the working practices of non-medical prescribers – for example, if a medicine is prescribed by a pharmacist independent prescriber, it should not be possible for the same pharmacist to perform a verify/clinical check on the order.

It is an important principle that a user's level of permissions to access records and use the system should be appropriate to their role. This is true for any business with client or customer responsibility, but is especially so for a healthcare setting, with the <u>duty of care</u> that health professionals have for their patients. Software vendors therefore need to ensure that datasets for <u>user permissions</u> are compliant with known <u>regional or national standards</u>. <u>Role-based access (RBAC)</u> is an important deliverable for a regional or national system, and was one of the aims of the English <u>Connecting for Health</u> program. One of the most important lessons concerning role based access was that the mapping of data items between the application database and the central data requirements was crucial for ensuring appropriate communications between systems, where concepts within the user permissions data locally may not be supported by <u>regional or national standards</u> for data and communications channels. Thus, it may not be possible to replicate all aspects of local user permissions in a national system.

Records Management and Multi-user Systems

An important issue arising from discussion of the risks associated with non-medical prescribing concerns the management of records within an EP system, where there may be multiple simultaneous users of the system.

This issue is essentially concerned with the system logic for record access within an EP system, and is not unique to the situation where a patient's prescribing record may be accessed by two or more prescribers simultaneously. System designers will need to consider the rules for record access and <u>record locking</u> for a variety of <u>multiuser system</u> scenarios. Rules would need to be applied to different levels of the system to ensure the smooth operation of the system. For example, it would be appropriate to lock a patient's prescribing record if a prescriber attempted to alter a dose of one medicine while a second prescriber was in the process of adding a new medicine to the prescribing profile. It would also be appropriate to lock a patient record if a pharmacist was attempting to verify/clinical check a <u>discharge prescription</u>, while a prescriber was in the process of adding another medicine to the <u>discharge prescription</u>. However, it would not be appropriate to lock a patient record if a nurse was administering a prescribed and checked medicine on a patient's profile, while a prescriber was in the process of adding a new medicine to the profile; this would impede the normal use of the system.

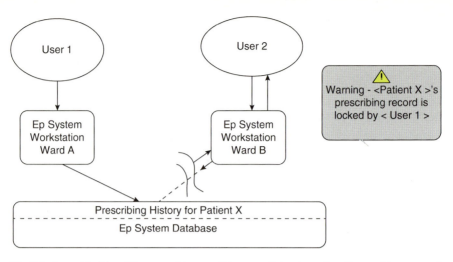

Fig. 7.1 Record locking. When user 1 is prescribing a medicine for patient X, user 2 is prevented from accessing the same patient record. User 2 will be warned that the record is in use by user 1 and will have read-only access to the record

If a record was locked against a second or subsequent user, a warning message would display, as shown in Fig. 7.1.

For two or more prescribers using the system simultaneously, it would be appropriate for the patient's record to be locked at the prescribing level for second and subsequent prescribers. This ensures that (a) the prescriber knows that they are viewing the full current <u>prescribing history</u> for a patient at the point where they are about to prescribe a new item, and (b) the second prescriber knows that another prescriber is in the process of prescribing for the patient. A useful feature would be for the <u>record locking</u> warning message to display the identity of the first prescriber to the second prescriber, to facilitate communications between prescribers of different types.

Once an item has been prescribed, consideration needs to be given to the time taken for all workstation screens to refresh with the amended prescribing record with the new item or amendment showing. This will depend on client-server communications in a networked system.

The other issue highlighted was that of access to prescribing records, and input of prescriptions by non-medical prescribers who may be <u>peripatetic healthcare professionals</u>. Electronic systems offer solutions to this problem, and there has been considerable experience of using portable devices for inputting medical information in peripatetic settings. Typically, a system might use a <u>slave application</u> mounted on a portable device, such as a <u>personal digital assistant (PDA)</u> or a <u>palm PC</u> or <u>tablet PC</u>. The slave application would have some, or all, of the functionality of the main system, together with a subset of patient records, depending on the memory capability of the device. The peripatetic health professional would enter the relevant patient information on the device and then, at some future time, the information on the device would be downloaded to the main application, either via a networked connection at the hospital or healthcare provider site, or via a telephone dial-up connection. This downloading process would also include the synchronization of the patient data on the portable device with the patient data on the main application.

This type of solution has been used for <u>clinical noting</u> by <u>peripatetic healthcare professionals</u> involved with <u>mental health</u> and <u>palliative care</u>, and could be used to facilitate EP functions. There are, however, a number of issues with the use of this approach with EP:

(a) EP requires a <u>drug database</u> to work from, and there may be problems with accessing a comprehensive drug database from a portable device. However, non-medical prescribers, even independent ones, are likely to be using a limited formulary within the context of a particular healthcare setting, which will reduce the size of the database required. Furthermore, certain care scenarios can be catered for by a small and well-defined set of prescriptions, perhaps available on the device as <u>pre-defined orders (PDOs)</u>.

(b) Because the portable device is not operating in real time, the <u>synchronization</u> of the slave application with the main system is of particular significance in EP application. If, at the point of synchronization, a prescriber is already using the main system, then the data transfer from the portable device should be locked in exactly the same way as would happen if a second user was using the main system. Because of the real time problem, there may also be issues with provision of <u>clinical checks</u> – e.g. drug interactions, duplicate therapy etc. The slave application cannot provide full <u>decision support</u> because it cannot view the full patient prescribing record. In any case, there may be issues with mounting data to provide prescribing decision support tools on the portable device. The decision support checking process would therefore need to take place retrospectively at the point of synchronization with the master system, when the "full" prescribing history is known to the master system (and probably using decision support routines mounted on the master system). There would therefore need to be a process of clinical warning messaging to the portable device, and perhaps a function whereby certain orders are automatically inactivated on the main application if there are serious drug interactions. Another approach – the most likely approach in practice – would be not to implement decision support functions and to reduce clinical risks by limiting the prescribing functions on the hand-held device.

Workflow for Different Prescriber Types

As has already been discussed, one of the benefits of an EP system to prescribers of all professional backgrounds is that it facilitates the generation of clear, complete and accurate prescriptions [13, 14]. This benefit is of value both to experienced prescribers who may be complacent about clarity and completeness of prescriptions, and also to newer prescribers from other healthcare professions, who may be inexperienced in the process of prescription writing. However, in addition to the standard prescribing workflow, consideration should be given to the specific needs and requirements for non-medical prescribers in the design of an EP system's <u>prescribing workflow</u>.

A number of extra factors in the prescribing process should be considered when designing an EP system to support non-medical prescribers.

Prescribing Permissions

For a user to be able to prescribe at all, they need the following attributes: (1) designation of a prescriber type under <u>user permissions</u>, and (2) current details of <u>professional accreditation</u>, <u>training</u> and <u>professional insurance</u> to be entered onto the system under user information.

Structured Prescribing and Care Plans

As mentioned, an important distinction within non-medical prescribers is between <u>dependent prescribers</u>, and <u>independent prescribers</u>. The former can only prescribe medicines for a patient within the context of an agreed <u>clinical management plan (CMP)</u> set up for that patient by an independent prescriber. In contrast, an independent prescriber can prescribe medicines for a patient independently of any <u>care plan</u> or pathway.

In practice, this would mean that there would be functionality in an EP system for an independent prescriber to set up a customized CMP for a patient, or to implement a standard locally-agreed care pathway for a specific patient. The CMP or care pathway would have embedded in it a series of orders, or an order set, which could subsequently be prescribed as a prescription by a dependent prescriber.

Therefore, on activating the prescribing function, an independent prescriber would have the option of prescribing for the patient directly from the system formulary, or setting up a CMP for the patient to be followed by a dependent prescriber. By contrast, when a dependent prescriber activates the prescribing function, any activated CMPs for the patient are displayed. If there are no valid CMPs set up for the patient, the dependent prescriber cannot proceed with the prescribing process for that patient. Each CMP will contain medicine orders, which can be activated by the dependent prescriber to generate prescriptions. It is likely that each CMP will have logic embedded in it possibly with limits to prescribing dependent on time, test results or other medicines prescribed. There may be certain situations where the dependent prescriber is forced to refer the CMP back to the independent prescriber, and can no longer proceed with implementing the care plan. Possible <u>prescribing workflows</u> for <u>non-medical prescribers</u> are illustrated in Fig. 7.2.

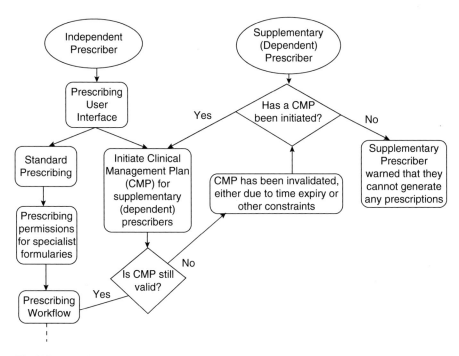

Fig. 7.2 Prescribing workflow for non-medical prescribers. NB the validation process may be iterative as there may be several CMPs set up for each supplementary prescriber at any one time

To facilitate prescribing by supplementary prescribers, EP systems will need to have a library of local and national CMPs or care pathways. Correspondingly, hospitals and healthcare providers will need to have a robust procedure for the design, set-up, validation and maintenance of the CMP/care pathway library, in just the same way as individual drug formulations and pre-defined orders (PDOs)/order sets (see Chap. 5).

Specialist Formularies

While, in the UK, nurse and pharmacist independent prescribers can, in theory, prescribe from a full formulary, the official recommendation is that they prescribe within their area of competence [15]. This recommendation, together with the need for healthcare providers to manage clinical risk and to control expenditure, will mean that independent prescribers working in the context of secondary care healthcare institutions will almost certainly be working with a specialist formulary. Depending on the work done by independent prescribers within an organization, the specialist formulary will either be for all independent prescribers within the organization, or there will be a specialist formulary for each specialty in the organization. Thus, on activating the prescribing function on the EP system, a non-medical independent prescriber will be able to select medicines from a specialist formulary, compiled for their use. It should be noted that, at this point, there may be little distinction between medical (independent) prescribers and non-medical independent prescribers; some implementers of EP systems have set up core and specialist formularies, which prevent junior medical staff from prescribing specialist treatments that are outside the specialty of their current rotation.

Information Support for Different Non-medical Prescriber Types

As mentioned previously, there is now much information on medicines that is available in electronic form. This may take the form of electronic versions of standard pharmaceutical compendia, such as the BNF and MIMS, or alternatively web-based information from specialist centers much as the Cochrane Centre, and the Medicines Resource Centre (MeReC). As well as published information, there are also local clinical guidelines and other local documentation, which may be on a hospital intranet or local network.

Resources such as these can easily be made available for prescribing decision support within an EP system, subject to licensing arrangements for the published sources. This is typically done in a passive format, where a button is put within the EP software allowing the user to access the referential information, if required, by pressing the button.

Referential information on medicines is of equal value to all types of prescriber, especially for those medicines where there are very specific criteria for use. However, given the usual mode of using reference information for passive decision support within EP systems, consideration should be given to implementation of more active decision support for non-medical prescribers. For supplementary prescribers, the CMP or care pathway can be a useful vehicle for information to support the prescribing process. For independent non-medical prescribers, however, there may be a case for presenting prescribing support information actively within the prescribing process. For example, if a nurse independent prescriber were to prescribe the single-dose fluconazole 150 mg capsule for a woman with vaginal candidiasis (thrush), an EP system would actively display current national or local clinical guidelines for thrush treatment as part of the prescribing workflow.

Support for Patient Group Directions (PGDs)

In the UK, a patient group direction (PGD) is a written protocol, enabling the supply of a medicine, or group of medicines, to patients who fit certain criteria, where the patients do not have to be individually identifiable in advance of the supply being made [16]. PGDs can legally be administered by a range of health professionals, including nurses, midwives, health visitors, optometrists, pharmacists, podiatrists, radiographers, orthoptists, physiotherapists, ambulance paramedics, dieticians, occupational therapists, prosthetists, orthotists and speech therapists [17]. Other countries have similar provisions for group protocol supply arrangements.

PGDs are of importance where a high volume of patients will present for a specific treatment, but it is unknown who will attend. They are typically used, therefore, to enable the supply of medicines in settings other than medical offices/surgeries, often in response to public health treatment needs. Examples of this are the supply of the antibiotic azithromycin for people with chlamydia infection at a <u>sexually transmitted diseases (STD) clinic</u>, or the supply of vaccines at a <u>travel clinic</u>.

While the use of a PGD is not a form of prescribing, it is a means by which a variety of health professionals might be involved with the supply of a medicine. It would be appropriate, therefore, for an EP system to be involved with the management of services involving PGDs in secondary care.

With PGDs or group protocols, the <u>business process</u> for medicine supply would centre on the PGD, rather than on the patient, and the part of the system dealing with PGDs would constitute a separate module to the system. Ideally, the system would provide a criteria checklist for the clinical user, attached to each PGD. This would enable the user to check that the presenting patient is eligible to be treated under the PGD, using similar functionality as for prospective clinical trial patients, as discussed in Chap. 6, and would form an <u>audit trail</u> for healthcare managers. Once eligibility has been established, the protocol treatment would be allocated to the patient, and a record of the treatment would be posted onto the prescribing record for the patient, if present within the system, and the user would be notified of any decision support warnings that arise (contraindications, interactions etc). System designers should consider the applicability of functionality to prevent sensitive <u>personal information</u> – for example, concerning the treatment of <u>HIV infection</u> and <u>sexually transmitted diseases</u> – from being visible on the general prescribing profile, which would be visible to a wide range of users in the healthcare organization and beyond, but still be listed in the physical record, and be available for decision support checking.

Support for Training and CPD for Non-medical Prescribers

As mentioned previously, one of the key risk areas highlighted in reviews of non-medical prescribing has been the <u>training</u> of non-medical prescribers. Given that all clinical professions have requirements for <u>continuing professional development (CPD)</u>, the issue of training is continuous with that of CPD, as a non-medical prescriber is usually learning prescribing skills in order to develop their professional practice. It should be pointed out that training and development of prescribing skills is an area that is not limited to non-medical prescribers; it would also be applicable to less experienced medical prescribers, such as foundation year doctors/interns.

Indeed, structured training on prescribing skills during the course of work experience would be a positive development for junior doctors in some areas.

The contribution that EP systems are able to make to the continuing professional development of healthcare professionals was discussed in the previous chapter. However, EP systems are able to facilitate the development of prescribing skills and knowledge in all professional groups involved with medicine prescribing. As mentioned earlier, EP systems could be configured so that non-medical prescribers benefit from more active decision support during the prescribing process.

The prescribing process on an EP system can be a useful source of information for professional development for prescribers from all disciplines and of all levels of experience. Sources of information for CPD would include Care Management Plans (CMPs), care pathways and clinical decision support warnings (drug interactions, sensitivities, precautions and contraindications), as long as they are implemented in a way that is clear, relevant and does not excessively impede the prescribing workflow.

Furthermore, there is the potential for EP systems to provide simulation training for less experienced prescribers. Such simulation might be active or passive. With passive simulated prescribing training, a particular workstation – preferably not in a clinical area – would be switched to draw patient data from a training database, to allow a user to practice their prescribing, using the EP software, but against dummy patients. The training database would need to be clearly identifiable as a non-live database.

A further advance would be the development of an active prescribing simulation module, whereby the EP system would automatically present the trainee prescriber with a specific patient and a clinical scenario, and the prescriber would then prescribe for the patient using the EP system. The system would then simulate a response – or lack of response – to treatment by the patient, in terms of clinical observations and test results fed back etc. The prescriber would then review the therapeutic strategy on the basis of the simulated patient response, and act accordingly. At the end of the simulation training session using the EP system, the system could then feed back to the trainee prescriber, with an evaluation of the decisions they made.

The development of an active simulation module within an EP system would constitute a highly sophisticated and potentially complex enhancement, especially if a large number of clinical scenarios were incorporated. Consequently, this represents a highly advanced function of future EP implementations. Nevertheless, active simulation would enable prescribers not only to develop their prescribing skills, but also to increase their knowledge of the EP system and its functions.

Adverse Drug Event (ADE) Reporting

Following the thalidomide issue in the late 1960s, it became commonplace for the pharmaceutical industry and healthcare providers to monitor new medicines to assess their safety in use, and to detect common adverse drug events (ADEs). In the UK, the Committee on Safety of Medicines (CSM) was set up in order to oversee this safety monitoring, or pharmacovigilance, process. Since then, pharmacovigilance has become an increasingly sophisticated science. However, while pharmaceutical manufacturers still collate adverse drug events from pre- and post-marketing clinical studies on their products, and recent regulatory changes have required pharmaceutical manufacturers to scan published literature for evidence of new ADEs, a key route for identifying ADEs has been spontaneous reporting by health professionals.

The CSM's Yellow Card Scheme was designed to encourage the spontaneous reporting of ADEs by doctors [18] when patients returned to the prescriber to report a side effect issue with a prescribed medicine. On being informed of a potential ADE by the patient, the prescriber completes a yellow card, which are distributed with prescription pads and copies of the British National Formulary, and sends the report to the CSM to be added to their database, either as a hard-copy yellow card form, or via the CSM yellow card website. The CSM reports regularly to pharmaceutical companies and also produces safety awareness bulletins.

It has long been acknowledged that the Yellow Card scheme detects only a proportion of the actual ADEs observed with a new medicine. Consequently, in 1999, the CSM expanded the Yellow Card reporting scheme to allow other healthcare professionals to report suspected ADEs, in an attempt to increase the detection power of the scheme. Then, in 2002, the CSM introduced a web-based electronic yellow card reporting tool for health professionals. However, despite both of these innovations, there is still considerable under-reporting of spontaneous ADEs through the yellow card scheme.

Nevertheless, EP systems clearly have a potential role in the processing of electronically reported ADEs by health professionals, subject to the availability of appropriate regulatory channels for the electronic ADE reporting in a particular healthcare economy. It has been suggested by UK commentators [19] and German commentators [20] that electronic ADE reporting via clinician workstations would lead to a significant increase in the numbers of spontaneous ADEs reported, simply because there would be an opportunity for the ADE data to be captured at the point of patient consultation. ADE data capture at the point of consultation would mean that more details of the ADE would be available at the outset, which would reduce the need for follow-up by pharmaceutical companies or regulatory bodies. Then, even if there were incomplete details of the ADE, and follow-up was required, the ADE record would exist and could be flagged for follow up. A study of an EP system in Canada [21] indicated that the system ensured that the indication of a prescribed medicine was recorded at the time of prescribing, which would ensure completeness of the prescribing record; the authors indicated that this could enable the use of EP systems for drug safety reporting.

The ways in which an EP system can be configured to collect and send electronic ADE reports will be a significant issue for future EP implementers, as well as for regulators, because of the growth in non-medical prescribing, together with the likelihood of increased use of EP systems by prescribers from other healthcare disciplines (which is why this issue is being considered under this chapter heading).

A possible process for electronic ADE reporting would be as follows:

(a) A healthcare professional (HCP) identifies an ADE in one of their patients.
(b) The HCP launches the ADE functionality of the EP system from whichever part of the EP system they are using (it would be important for the ADE functionality of an EP system to be accessed from many different parts of the EP system, in order to facilitate a high degree of ADE data capture).
(c) The ADE form would be launched. A patient identifier would be populated automatically (anonymized from the PAS).
(d) The HCP would be required to select which of the patient's current medications was implicated in the ADE. The system should allow selection of two or three suspect drugs. Selection in this way would allow the ADE form to be coded with the drug details.
(e) Using the coded drug details, there would then be an option for the HCP to view the known side effects of the suspect drugs for information.
(f) The HCP would then complete other ADE details – ADE type (MEDDRA code or other relevant code), ADE outcome (MEDDRA code or other relevant code), concomitant medication, and additional details.
(g) The reporter details (and clinician details, if different) would be supplied from the user database.
(h) If necessary, the ADE would then be flagged up to the attending doctor to be validated before transmission. In some countries, this might be a legal requirement; in others, it may be a convention for the healthcare provider organization involved. However, it should be borne in mind that, if clinician validation is a prerequisite to submission of the ADE report, the number of reports submitted might be artificially limited, and ADEs may be lost to follow up.
(i) Once the ADE report has been sent, the details would need to be retained within the EP system database, with a unique identifier. Then, if the regulatory body or pharmaceutical company wanted to follow up the ADE report, to obtain further information, then the follow up could take place. This might be by a message to the EP system, triggering reactivation of the ADE record, or by an e-mail to the reporter, advising them to update the ADE record and resubmit it.

The functionality described here represents advanced EP functionality, and there are many potential barriers to its implementation. These include lack of agreement between the various stakeholders in both the regulatory and the healthcare sectors concerning data standards and reporting conventions, the organizational capacity of regulators to process the increased amount of ADE information that it might receive, and the likelihood that EP systems suppliers will incorporate such functionality into their systems in an appropriate and useable manner. Above all, there still remains the inertia of health professionals in reporting ADEs in the first place, despite the use of electronic systems to facilitate the process.

European regulatory bodies are working on a common dataset to allow the transmission of ADE data from pharmaceutical companies to licensing authorities. Over the last few years, there has been an initiative where the European electronic ADE dictionary, MEDDRA, has been made available free to healthcare provider bodies [22], which would provide the data support for electronic ADR reporting.

Non-medical Prescribing: Management and Clinical Governance

One of the advantages of all electronic systems is that they capture data on the <u>business processes</u> that they are designed to automate. Consequently, it is possible to extract data from these applications in order to manage and evaluate the business processes taking place. This may be to provide an <u>audit trail</u> – to ensure that the process is taking place in the way that it should, and that system users are working within their occupational roles. Alternatively, this data extraction may be to provide <u>management reports</u>, to show that levels of service are being met, to monitor the system throughput and to highlight areas of concern.

<u>Management reporting</u> and <u>audit trails</u> are an area of particular concern in prescribing and medicines management, where both standards of professional practice and the need to deliver <u>health outcomes</u> against costs are important drivers. General issues associated with management reporting from EP systems are discussed elsewhere in this book. However, it is important to note that the reporting and audit trail functions of an EP system have a particular role in management, training and service development of services and clinics led by non-medical prescribers.

One of the issues highlighted in publications on non medical prescribing is that, at present, there is very little comparative data on the prescribing patterns of different professional groups [1] and, now that nurse and pharmacist <u>independent prescribers</u> are established, there is a pressing need for these data, in order to evaluate services provided and the <u>skill mix</u> required to provide them. The establishment of EP systems that support the activities of non-medical prescribers provide the environment from which, in theory, such comparative data can be extracted. Nevertheless, as with reporting from electronic systems in general, there are some important caveats with the use of EP systems to provide management reports on prescribing patterns for different types of prescriber. These include (a) ensuring that prescribing data extracts for different prescriber groups are comparable; (b) ensuring that the <u>user permissions</u> dataset is structured in an appropriately granular manner to allow different prescriber types and details to be extracted reliably.

Conclusion

As a result of changes in service level targets, health professional availability and societal attitudes, there is a need for optimal use of "skill mix" within healthcare provider organizations. That is to say, all staff should be working to their maximum capability to enable the most effective service provision within the organization. There is therefore a rationale for healthcare professionals other than doctors to take responsibility for prescribing in certain areas (for example, in specialty areas, or those where other professionals will have a greater knowledge of the products than doctors (e.g. dressings and dietary products)). For this reason, prescribing by other professional groups is on the increase in countries around the world. EP systems have a number of benefits for a "mixed economy" of prescribers. They ensure that system access levels and prescribing processes are appropriate to each type of prescriber. Furthermore, EP systems are able to maintain records of training and accreditation for non-medical prescribers, and to provide support to different prescribers in terms of information support and continuing professional development resources.

References

1. Anon. Non-medical prescribing. Drug Ther Bull. 2006;44:33–7.
2. Latter S, Courtenay MJ. Effectiveness of nurse prescribing: a review of the literature. J Clin Nurs. 2004;13:26–32.
3. Capper E, Jones SW. Are patients satisfied with a pharmacist-led rheumatology drug monitoring clinic? Pharm J. 1999;263:R66.
4. Tadros LBM, Ledger-Scott M, et al. The pharmacist-led diabetic scheme improves glycaemic control in insulin-requiring type 2 diabetic patients. Int J Pharm Pract. 2003;11:R14.
5. Latter S, et al. An evaluation of extended formulary independent nurse prescribing. Executive summary of final report. University of Southampton, Department of Health. 2005.
6. General Medical Council. An in-depth investigation into causes of prescribing errors by foundation trainees in relation to their medical education — EQUIP study. 2009. http://www.dh.gov.uk/en/Publicationsandstatistics/Publications/PublicationsPolicyAndGuidance/DH_4071443. Accessed in May 2012.
7. Audit Commission. A spoonful of sugar: medicines management in NHS hospitals. London: Audit Commission; 2001.
8. Smith J, editor. Building a safer NHS for patients: improving medication safety. London: Department of Health; 2004.
9. Committee on Safety of Medicines. Summary of the Committee on Safety of Medicines Meeting held on Thursday 27th October, 2005.
10. McVeigh FL. E-prescribing in optometry practice. Optometry. 2008;79:692–701.
11. Slee A. E-prescribing in Birmingham. Presented at the Guild of Healthcare Pharmacists/United Kingdom Clinical Pharmacy Association Information Technology Interest Group (ITIG) seminar. Birmingham, UK. 2010. http://www.ghp.org.uk/ContentFiles/ghpitig10a.pps
12. Niazkhani Z, Pirnejad H, et al. Computerised provider order entry system – does it support the interprofessional medication process? Lessons from a Dutch academic hospital. Methods Inf Med. 2010;49:20–7.
13. Farrar K. Accountability, prescribing and hospital pharmacy in an electronic, automated age. Pharm J. 1999;263:496–501.
14. Farrar K. In: Smith J, editors. Building a safer NHS for patients: improving medication safety. London: Department of Health. 2004. p. 128.
15. Improving patients' access to medicines: a guide to implementing nurse and pharmacist independent prescribing within the NHS in England. London: Department of Health. 2005. http://www.dh.gov.uk/assetRoot/04/13/37/47/04133747.pdf
16. Patient Group Directions. A practical guide and framework of competencies for all professionals using patient group directions. Liverpool: National Prescribing Centre; 2004.
17. Anon. Non-medical prescribing. Drug Ther Bull. 2006;44:34.
18. Committee on Safety of Medicines. About the yellow card scheme. 1999; 12th November:3–4.
19. Reporting Adverse Drug Reactions. A guide for healthcare professionals. London: British Medical Association; 2006.
20. Thurmann PA. Methods and systems to detect adverse drug reactions in hospitals. Drug Saf. 2001;24:961–8.
21. Equale T, Winslade N, et al. Enhancing pharmacosurveillance with systematic collection of treatment indication in electronic prescribing: a validation study in Canada. Drug Saf. 2010;33:559–67.
22. Anon. Dictionary for ADR reporting to be free for healthcare providers. PIPA J. 2007;15:21.

Chapter 8
Electronic Prescribing and Future Priorities

As mentioned in the introduction, this book is not intended as an exhaustive review of EP research; rather, it is designed to help EP implementers and stakeholders to reflect on the various methodological, clinical and professional issues associated with electronic prescribing. The previous chapters have aimed to do this from the standpoint of a number of recognized benefit areas of EP systems. This final chapter is therefore arguably the most speculative chapter, as it aims to consider the future challenges and areas of development in EP implementation.

Many of the areas of innovation described here are very advanced, considering the proportion of healthcare providers in the UK and the US with EP systems, and the level of functionality provided by those EP systems. However, tender documents and output-based specifications (OBS) often consist of "blue skies" wish-lists of possible future EP functions, often compiled by idealistic clinicians and managers, with no implementation experience, and it is worth exploring the possibility of some of these proposed functions.

Nevertheless, as a general rule, many implementers recognize the importance of implementing basic EP functions well within a hospital or healthcare provider, before enhancing the system to provide more advanced functions. It is recognized that EP systems are sociotechnical systems, which evolve with use, and that even basic functionality should be considered "work in progress" and should be monitored for any unintended clinical consequences [1].

While this chapter cites some of the literature on emerging technologies which may have EP applications, it should be noted that these comments are made in the light of the author's experience across a range of medicines management IT applications.

The Challenge of Device Integration

As has been discussed in previous chapters, the interfacing of EP systems with other applications – in particular patient administration systems (PAS) and pharmacy systems – is desirable in order to promote the intraoperability of systems, and thus a

S. Goundrey-Smith, *Principles of Electronic Prescribing*, Health Informatics,   155
DOI 10.1007/978-1-4471-4045-0_8, © Springer-Verlag London 2012

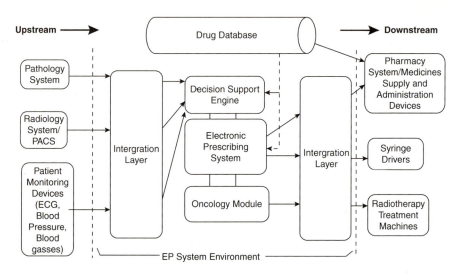

Fig. 8.1 Device integration upstream and downstream of the prescribing process. Upstream integrations are concerned with decision support and downstream integrations are concerned with medicine supply and delivery

seamless workflow for the user. As discussed, a seamless workflow promotes organizational efficiency and reduces risks associated with the rekeying of prescription data or the prescription data not being available to all users in real time. Therefore, an EP system should draw its patient demographic data from the PAS, take a feed from the pathology system for test results and then transmit any medicine orders placed directly to the pharmacy system, which may also have an ongoing interface with a pharmacy robot.

The interfaces described above are established requirements with many EP implementations, and have been delivered in various different ways in different installations and with different products. However, an area as yet to be fully explored is that of interfaces or integration with other devices. The terms *interface* and *integration* are both used here, but they are not synonymous. In this context, *interface* is used to describe a data link between two stand-alone software applications, to enable the intraoperability of the two applications. *Integration* describes how a device, which may have limited operating software of its own, is linked into another system, which not only channels data to and from the device, but also provides the software routines to control and drive the device. The device thus becomes an integral part of the bigger system.

The point of interface or integration may be upstream from the prescribing workflow – monitoring devices, especially in the intensive care unit scenario – or downstream from the prescribing workflow – devices to facilitate therapy or drug delivery (Fig. 8.1).

Device integration upstream of the prescribing process generally has as its goal the facilitation of clinical decision support. It is recognized that decision support tools are an essential aspect of any EP system [2], and that decision support applications have been in use in the United States to support prescribing well before the widespread introduction of computerized ordering of medicines (CPOE) [3]. However, as discussed in Chap. 5, decision support tools require accurate input information, in order to give an appropriate clinical warning to the user. Many decision support functionalities that have been developed thus far in EP systems – for example, drug interactions, duplicate therapy and drug doubling checking – are internally referential, as they use data that are already within the drug database of an EP system; data that are relatively static. Other decision support functions – such as sensitivity checking, contraindications and drug-disease warnings – rely on data from systems that are external to the EP system, usually data fields that are attached to the patient record on the PAS. These functions are more problematic because, although these data too are relatively static, there are potential issues with the currency of the patient-related data on a PAS record, with the effective transmission of that data between the PAS and the EP system, and with conflict between data values stored in two different locations.

For example, an EP system may have links with a pathology system, or with a radiology system, with order communications and picture archiving computer system (PACS) functions. Many hospitals currently provide ward access to pathology systems, so that clinicians can review test results prior to prescribing drugs, or amending drug doses. Electronic access to pathology system test ordering and results review functionality, along with EP functions, as part of an integrated clinical workstation is already a reality for some healthcare providers. However, it is to be hoped that in future there would be a direct data pull from a pathology system in order to facilitate the prescribing of certain drugs. For example, whenever a diuretic is prescribed, the system will automatically retrieve the latest potassium result from the pathology system, and display it (together with the date that the sample was taken) on the prescribing screen. There could also be the option for the prescriber to order new U&E tests from the prescribing screen. As well as specific monitoring tests for individual drugs (for example, electrolytes with diuretics, or hematology results (hemoglobin, serum iron etc) for anemia treatments), there is the possibility of a batch feed of antibiotic susceptibilities to support a more complex decision support module for antibiotic prescribing (see Chap. 4).

Also, it is to be hoped that, eventually, hardware advances (monitor resolution enhancements) will allow an EP user to access radiology system functions and PACS on the same workstation as the EP system. However, full integration of PACS facilities into an EP system may be technically difficult and, in any case, with the possible exception of an oncology system where images are required for tumor staging, may not be a high priority, compared to some other integration requirements.

However, while the integrations described above can improve the prescribing decision support process, the logical goal of clinical decision support in electronic prescribing is a system that provides decision support intuitively, working with dynamic data from patient monitoring devices, such as blood pressure and blood gas monitoring devices.

In general terms, the EP software would respond to variations in dynamic monitoring data – for example, threshold or out-of-range triggers – and send a warning to the clinical user, either on screen on the application, or routed via a pager or SMS text message, advising them of the therapeutic options for the patient. In some care situations, especially critical care scenarios where the EP system was linked downstream to a syringe driver, it would be desirable for the EP system to make automatic dose adjustments, based on monitoring results.

Device integration downstream of the prescribing process is generally concerned with the automated scheduling and delivery of treatment to the patient. A standard example of this is the integration of a syringe driver with an EP system. Syringe drivers are devices that deliver injectable medicines from a syringe at a set rate of infusion. The device is programmable with the required infusion rate, and can detect blockages in the line and other interruptions to the flow rate. Syringe drivers with highly sophisticated control mechanisms are often referred to in the literature as "smart" pumps. However, it has been determined [4] that smart pump technology alone is unlikely to reduce medication errors without:

(a) interface with an EP system, or an electronic patient record (EPR) system
(b) barcode based medicines administration functionality
(c) pharmacy information systems

Integration of a syringe pump with an EP system would enable, for example, a patient on a intensive care unit to be given a continuous infusion of isosorbide dinitrate injection in a Graseby type syringe driver, driven by an EP system. Then, when the patient's heart rate changes, a warning message would be sent to a prescriber. The prescriber would adjust the infusion rate on the electronic administration profile of the EP system (possibly remotely), and the infusion rate would be automatically changed on the syringe driver.

Another area where there is established experience of integration with medical devices is in the field of oncology systems. Cancer treatment protocols are increasingly mixed-modality in their format; that is to say that a particular protocol for the treatment of a certain type of cancer might consist in total of some cycles of chemotherapy and some cycles of radiotherapy. Thus, in recent years, there has been an increasing need for oncology clinic management systems to be interfaced with radiotherapy treatment equipment, so that the clinic management software can schedule and deliver radiotherapy treatment as well as chemotherapy treatments. There are therefore a number of oncology systems that offer interfaces and integration with radiotherapy treatment machines. In some of these cases, clinic management software is developed as an add-on to the device control software, and this may not be satisfactory for providing full oncology prescribing functionality. In other cases, device integration is provided as part of a comprehensive suite of oncology clinic software. However, in either case, the fact remains that radiotherapy device integration expertise has been gained specifically within oncology management software and it may not be easy for software vendors to develop radiotherapy device integration within the context of a comprehensive general EP solution.

Other downstream device integrations might include integration with pharmacy systems, and integration with ward-based medicine storage devices. Such integrations are designed to ensure the accurate and safe delivery of the medicine that has been prescribed. A number of EP systems have already been implemented with a link to the pharmacy system, with the data mapping issues that such a link entails.

This integration enables the automatic ordering of medicines from the pharmacy and the seamless pharmaceutical supply chain, with the organizational benefits that it provides (see Chap. 3). A step further would be the integration of an EP system, with a pharmacy system *and* a pharmacy robot, as this would facilitate automated, bar-code mediated [1] product picking at the pharmacy. Because of potential mapping issues with the data for each of the three systems, there is an argument for running the three systems from a single database platform. So, for example, if a comprehensive third-party drug database, mounted on a central server location, could be used as the data platform for all three applications, various technical issues associated with data mapping between the systems would be resolved.

As well as facilitating the electronic ordering and supply of medicines using pharmacy system and robot interfaces upstream of the prescribing process, an EP system may also be integrated with medicine dispensing devices, such as ward-based electronic medicine dispensing cabinets (so-called "magic cupboards"), and electronic drug trolleys [5]. In this way, the EP system will have close control over the medicine administration process.

By the integration of devices into the EP system in this way, decision support and monitoring processes for medicine use can be made automatic, closed loop processes in just the same way that the diagnosis, prescribing and supply processes can be. Device integration, however, presents a number of major challenges to the advanced development of EP systems:

(a) The ability of EP software vendors to keep up with developments in medical device technology and produce appropriate interface and control routines for the devices that are in current use.
(b) The use of appropriate system algorithms for device control and data feeds.
(c) The development of appropriate data standards to support intraoperability between different device types.

Various larger software vendors have conducted some work on device integration but many of the interfaces and software routines developed are only at the prototype stage. The universal clinical use of a range of device interfaces in hospitals and healthcare provider organizations is still very much in the future, with the exception of centers where there is in-house healthcare informatics expertise, and a proven record of healthcare IT innovation.

Smart Packaging

Work has also been conducted to develop systems for smart packaging of medicines [6]. Smart packaging typically resembles a standard medicine blister pack, but contains a microchip that can record the time each dose is removed from the packaging. These packs can also provide anti-tamper functions, record storage conditions and

---

[1] However, it should be remembered that not every product has a barcode attached to it. There may be problems with mapping across all three systems.

monitor symptom/side effect scores from patients. Worldwide data standards now exist to record and transmit data from these devices and so there is now the possibility to interface them with EP systems, in order to provide compliance and side-effect monitoring as part of the EP process. However, there are a number of difficult issues relating to this. Firstly, there are ethical issues associated with the process. Patients would need to consent to the data being collected on their medicine-taking behavior; some patients might feel that this is intrusive, or might not want the data shared with all healthcare personnel. Secondly, this would only be a secondary test of compliance; the patient might take the tablet or capsule out of the package, but might not ingest the medicine. Thirdly, the accuracy of any monitoring data will depend on the controls on the smart packaging and the design of any underlying algorithm.

Hardware Platforms and Infrastructure

Improvements in available hardware technology have impacted on EP system configuration. The earliest EP/CPOE systems consisted of a specific medicines management module of a hospital information system (HIS), which was usually configured as a series of terminals connected to a mainframe computer via a physical local area network (LAN). Systems were subsequently developed on a client-server architecture, but still with a physical network connection.

While many such configurations provided adequate system performance for both EP order communication and decision support querying, the hardware was less than ideal for a clinical setting, consisting of large, cumbersome workstations, with a physical connection to each machine. Such hardware was not easily moveable, and the physical wiring had the potential to be a danger to staff. Most notably, it was difficult to structure such hardware around the operational environment, which is an important prerequisite for a successful EP implementation. Impractical hardware is one reason why clinical professionals may be ambivalent about EP implementation, and why systems may be unpopular at the outset, until actual benefits are demonstrated.

The development of smaller computers – laptop PCs and devices such as tablet PCs – together with wireless networks, have enabled workstations to become more portable, and thus support more clinical activities. The use of wireless workstations has enabled the development of electronic medicines administration, and allowed clinicians to prescribe medicines electronically while on the ward round.

There are, however, disadvantages and other considerations with these developments. While obviating the need for cumbersome cable connections, wireless networks have given rise to concerns about:

(a) network coverage. Early implementers found that, due to the design of some old hospital buildings, wireless networks might have "cold spots" with no network coverage, which would interfere with the operation of the EP system.
(b) network security. Without appropriate security measures, EP system data transmitted by wireless network could be accessed by unauthorized users. Since much of this data is relating to specific patients, this would constitute a confidentiality issue.

Also, while smaller, more portable devices offer the potential for fast functionality at the point of care, there are disadvantages with their use. Firstly, the smallest devices, such as personal digital assistants (PDAs), do not have a screen that is large enough and provides the necessary resolution for on-screen electronic medicines administration. Secondly, such machines are subject to wear and tear and damage due to spillage and knocks in the clinical environment. There is therefore the argument that, instead of using laptop PCs and tablet PCs, which are relatively expensive, durable workstations or thin client configurations should be used.

Consequently, implementers have looked to different device modalities to provide the right balance of functionality and durability in the clinical environment. Some of the earlier freestanding devices were very cumbersome, often with a battery pack that was heavy, yet which had a limited life. However, recent use of tablet PCs, with software mounted in a thin client configuration, has provided an inexpensive user interface, with an appropriate screen for medicines administration.

It is to be hoped that, in future, there will be development of portable hardware, specifically designed for EP applications, which will fully facilitate the prescribing and medicines administration process in a near patient manner. PDAs are in routine use for other medical applications – most notably, clinical decision support, provision of reference information and clinical noting. Indeed, some clinical professionals use PDAs to support prescribing of medicines and to monitor medical treatment. While a PDA screen is too small to be used for electronic medicines administration, there is considerable potential for using PDAs for certain EP functions [7] – for example, monitoring functions, clinical noting for drug-related observations or decision support alerting functions [8].

Telecare

Most of the technology described in the previous section is concerned with streamlining the patient care processes in hospital, and enhancing professional practice. However, an important aspect of modern healthcare is the centrality of the patient in their treatment. As mentioned in earlier chapters, there has been a paradigm shift in the philosophy of healthcare in recent decades, which has been characterized by a number of factors:

(a) the consumerization of medicine, where governments and health agencies are actively encouraging patients to exercise choice in their medical care, including the choices of therapy and practitioners.

(b) the diminishing paternalism of the medical profession, together with the rise in the autonomy and importance of other health professionals in service delivery, most notably nurses.

(c) the rise in personalized medicine where the use of IT to automate processes can provide medical care that is customized to the individual patient, thus optimizing the quality of care.

There have been many publications describing the role of the "empowered patient" in twenty-first century healthcare. In England, the Connecting for Health program sought to embody the principle of patient choice – for example, in the "Choose and Book" appointment booking system. This is likely to continue in future, with the concept of "No choice about me, without me" underpinning NHS reform since 2010 [9], and the recent proposals to improve patient access to electronic medical records [10].

It is clear that a significant area where patients can and should have a greater degree of autonomy, and play an active part in their own care is in the management of chronic diseases. As discussed previously, it is recognized on both sides of the Atlantic that chronic diseases – such as diabetes, asthma and hypertension – are a major cause of increased patient morbidity and reduced quality of life, and therefore are a significant economic burden to the healthcare system. Such diseases are often treated with drugs whose role and pharmacological properties are well-established, but which require regular monitoring, and the most significant factor in the cost of these diseases is the cost of hospitalization and acute treatment for a patient whose disease has become uncontrolled.

American commentators have identified the huge potential of EP systems to contribute to evidence-based medicine in patients with chronic diseases [11]. However, at the current time, in the US, EP systems are used in a small proportion of acute hospitals. There is therefore very little experience, if any at all, in the use of secondary care EP systems to gather monitoring data for patients with chronic diseases, either from GP systems (primary care systems) or from remote devices. This is a potentially major area of expansion for secondary care EP systems. There is the possibility that a healthcare provider based EP system might become the "hub" for care of chronic diseases in a series of patient populations in the community – for example, diabetes, asthma or hypertension, as shown in Fig. 8.2.

Appropriate technology – such as the internet, digital televisions and mobile phones would be used to support and enable the patient, as they take responsibility for their day-to-day self-care at home and in the community. Healthcare IT researchers have identified the potential of the electronic health record as a means of empowering the patient and supporting care process involvement [12, 13].

Examples of telecare technology would include the following:

• Use of a mobile phone to submit blood glucose readings to a diabetes care module of an EP system. Warnings concerning the amendment of the monitoring schedule or the insulin regimen would then be automatically calculated and sent back to the patient via SMS text message.
• Use of a digital television in the patient's home to allow the patient to log on to patient monitoring web facilities to view graphical monitoring information on their disease.

While telecare to enable patients to manage chronic diseases might, at first sight, appear to be a form of device integration, assistive technology involves a wider range of device modalities and manufacturers than might be found in the acute clinical

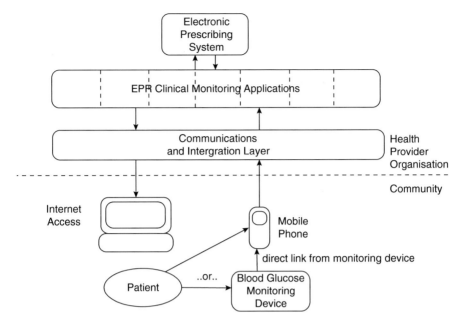

Fig. 8.2 EP and hospital information systems as a hub for patient self-management of chronic diseases

environment. Consequently, research in this area involves the coordination of a variety of stakeholders and is much more in its infancy, compared to system integration within the acute sector.

The remainder of this section will review literature which has evaluated telecare applications for the management of chronic diseases. Telecare services of different types have now been established in a range of therapeutic areas, including stroke [14], respiratory diseases [15, 16], remote intensive care unit (ICU) operation [17], palliative care [18, 19], obstetrics [20] and cardiovascular diseases [21, 22]. In some of these areas, evaluations have shown clear outcome benefits with the use of certain telecare services. Telecare has been shown to reduce rates of hospital admission in patients with asthma [15] and COPD [16]. In their study of patients with hypertension, Verberk et al. [21] showed that the use of a telecare service led to greater reductions in blood pressure than with conventional care, possibly due to a reduction in a "white coat" hypertension effect. Furthermore, in a study of remote ICU operation using telecare applications, Young et al. [17] found that the use of telecare applications to enable clinicians to access the ICU was associated with lower mortality levels in the ICU, and reduced length of stay in the ICU, probably because telecare enables more rapid clinician response than conventional care, if clinicians are not present at the time of critical incidents.

However, while studies have shown some clear outcome benefits with some forms of telecare, the benefits are not proven in all scenarios. Reviews of telecare in heart failure patients [22], obstetrics [20] and diabetes [23] have commented on the equivocal nature of the results in these areas. These and various other studies call for further research in telecare applications to determine further outcome benefits, to determine the exact patient profiles that would benefit from these services, and to provide data that are more robust from a study design perspective. In addition, some reviews have called for a more detailed cost-benefit analysis of telecare services [15, 24–26].

Notwithstanding the impact of telecare on outcome benefits, it is clear from the literature that telecare has considerable potential for improving personalized medicine, extending access to care and improving care access to patients in isolated situations. Telemedicine is beneficial in patients with poor mobility, such as spinal cord injuries and disorders [27], elderly and housebound patients [28] or those for whom the optimum care setting is their own home, such as palliative care patients [18]. Telecare modalities will also provide the basis for services that enable more patients to be treated without attending hospital – for example, outpatient parenteral antibiotics [29].

A number of studies have been conducted with the use of telemedicine software on mobile phones to help patients with the management and monitoring of chronic diseases [30], such as asthma and diabetes (Anhoj et al. [31], Farmer et al. [32]). These applications provided the advantage of real time uploading of monitoring information, and therefore in theory, a more accurate record of patient response to therapy. However, in these studies, the display of monitoring data on the phone screen was difficult to read for patients.

Gammon et al. [33] studied the use of a system which transferred the blood glucose results for a child, from the child's blood glucose testing device to a parent's mobile phone. The aim of the study was to conduct a preliminary assessment of the feasibility and use of the system, and the study was conducted with a group of 15 young people, between 9 and 15 years of age. The system was found to be easy to use, but its value was primarily as a means of reassurance for the parents; issues arose with the system concerning the independence and autonomy of the young person, and their attitude to parental control. Young people who were good at monitoring their blood glucose levels found that, with the system, the number of parental reminders was reduced, because the parents had evidence of the child's compliance with the monitoring requirement. As might be expected, for children who were less reliable at monitoring their blood glucose, the use of the system increased the number of parental interventions. The authors commented, however, that increased parental monitoring did not necessarily lead to improved glycemic control, since it often led to conflict between the parent and the child, which had a negative effect on monitoring compliance.

Telecare has the potential to provide considerable benefits to well-motivated patients who are committed to monitoring their chronic diseases, and to the healthcare professionals that support them. In particular, real-time monitoring information feeds from stand-alone testing devices, or domiciliary telemedicine monitoring systems have the potential to contribute to decision support functions in EP systems both in the hospital and in the community. The interface of such systems with hospital EP systems, so that hospital clinicians can obtain a clear and reliable record of recent monitoring results (e.g. <u>blood glucose readings</u> with diabetes), may enable patients to be treated more efficiently in hospital for complications or relapses of their chronic diseases.

There are a number of barriers to adoption of telemedicine systems. They are as follows:

1. Lack of a generic dataset. A feature of many telemedicine prototypes is that their datasets are proprietary, and are specific to a particular device manufacturer. Work has recently been conducted on the development of a generic dataset, based on XML messaging, which can be used for a variety of devices and applications [34].
2. The willingness of stakeholders to cooperate in system development. The development of such systems, together with their prototyping and testing, will require close collaboration between a wide range of stakeholders, including clinical professionals, health informatics specialists, hospital IM&T professionals, together with software and hardware/device vendors.
3. The availability of funding for telecare services and the availability of appropriate evidence to support business cases to secure funding. These issues are being addressed by the current literature available but, as discussed, further work is needed on the cost-effectiveness issues.
4. The adoption of such modalities by patients and clinical professionals. As discussed in Chap. 1, it is recognized that there is an adoption curve to a change or innovation. Depending on personality and worldviews, some individuals will embrace a change of procedure willingly, whereas others will be reluctant. Indeed, the greater the potential impact on a new technology on a patient's personal life – and a near-patient telemedicine monitoring system can have a potentially major impact on a patient's way of life – the more information and reassurance a patient will need to adopt a new technology or procedure. Patient attitudes to disease and illness will also be a factor. Some patients will not want to be "empowered" in the treatment of their illness; they would rather be passive and leave responsibility for treatment with a healthcare professional.
5. Ethical issues associated with these technologies. The ethical issues with "smart" packaging would also, to some extent, apply to telecare; patients would need to give explicit consent for data to be collected, if it was not obvious that this was happening, and some patients might not want their data to be shared with other healthcare professionals. Telecare also raises ethical questions concerning the cost-effectiveness of service provision with expensive telecare modalities, the disengagement of patients from healthcare professionals as a result of telemedicine and how this affects clinical practice, and the suitability of systems for different patient groups (for example, children and the elderly)

Clinical Homecare

Related to telecare, where clinical consultation, diagnosis and disease monitoring may be provided directly to the patient's home via video and telecommunications technology, is clinical homecare, where a treatment is provided to the patient in their own home (either self-administered or administered by a health professional as part of the service). Clinical homecare is now widespread in the UK and US, and provides significant benefits in provision of therapy without the costs of outpatient or day case hospital attendance, and delivery of care in a way that is convenient and more acceptable to patients. However, it is a complex discipline requiring input from several stakeholders, typically an acute healthcare provider, a pharmaceutical company and the homecare company that actually delivers the therapy service. For this reason, the regulatory requirements are complicated – a homecare provider company may be simultaneously a registered pharmacy, a pharmaceutical manufacturer and a nursing care provider, and would need to comply with the relevant regulations [35]. Because of multiple stakeholders in homecare services and the use of different homecare companies for different services even by the same healthcare provider organization, a recent England Department of Health (DH) review has highlighted issues concerning the transparency of commissioning processes, a need for more robust governance by clinical leads in provider organizations and more regional coordination [36].

EP systems have the potential to support commissioning and governance of homecare services, if there are appropriate interfaces with homecare company IT systems and information systems to support commissioning. The England DH review has indicated that links with EP systems and standard pharmacy management systems are required to optimize homecare services [37].

Identification and Communications Technologies

An EP system with decision support tools, full electronic medicine administration functions and an interface with the hospital pharmacy system is likely to lead to a considerable reduction in the risks associated with the prescribing and administration of medicines in hospitals, in particular the risks associated with the selection of a medicine, the dissemination and fulfillment of the order, and the clarity of the administration instructions.

However, the use of identification technologies – optical barcodes and radio-frequency identification (RFID) technology – can further reduce the risk associated with medicine administration, by closing the loop of the medicine administration process. The ideal medicine administration scenario would therefore involve verifying both the identity of the patient and the identity of the drug to be administered. The patient's barcode on their wrist-band is scanned and the patient's identity would be checked against the patient record on the EP system, where the demographic data are usually retrieved from the hospital <u>PAS</u>. When the identity of the patient had been confirmed, the identity of the medicine to be administered is then confirmed by scanning the <u>barcode</u> on the medicine pack before a dose of the medicine is administered to the patient.

The EP implementation at Charing Cross Hospital, London, UK [5], used barcode identification of patients. At each <u>medicine administration event</u>, the EP system required the patient's barcode to be scanned, in order for the patient's drawer on the <u>electronic drug trolley</u> to be released, so that the nurse could access the patient's medication. This barcode patient identification function caused the percentage of occasions where the patient identity was not checked to be reduced from 82.6% to 18.9%. However, system compliance was limited by practices such as sticking the patient's barcode to their bedside cupboard, rather than to their wristband.

<u>Barcodes</u> are used for medicine identification by automated dispensing systems (<u>pharmacy robots</u>) [38], and within the pharmacy <u>procurement</u> process [39]. However, there is little documented experience of the use of medicine identification using barcodes in the context of EP system medicines administration at ward level. There are two main problems with the use of barcodes for medicine identification at the point of administration:

1. It is recognized that a small proportion (<10%) of medicinal products are not barcoded [40], for example, some specialist medicines, <u>parallel imports</u> and hospital repackaged medicines. This continues to be a barrier to universal use of barcodes for medicines administration in secondary care.
2. Barcode medicine identification relies on original barcoded packs being used for medicine administration at ward level. While this may be the norm in some countries, it is not routinely the case in the UK, although 28 day dispensing has had a positive impact on the use of original packs at ward level in UK hospitals.

In due course, optical barcodes will be superseded by radiofrequency identification (RFID) technologies [41], where an item is identified by a radio frequency emitting tag. While this technology avoids the cumbersome and intrusive use of <u>barcode scanners</u>, which may be an advantage in the clinical environment, it is subject to the same issues that might arise with other <u>wireless network</u> technologies. These include (a) security of data transmission; (b) reliability of data transmission, given the geographical features of hospital buildings, and (c) collision of data with data in other wireless networks.

While optical barcodes are not routinely in use for near-patient clinical applications "in the UK", the use of RFID technologies for these applications is even further in the future. A major issue in the adoption of these identification technologies is the harmonization of codes to allow their universal use at an international level. There is an initiative by the healthcare industries to standardize barcodes [41], but the process is slow, and there is the danger that optical barcode technology will be obsolete by the time any international standard has been achieved, and that there will be no coherent standardization strategy for RFID tagging. Nevertheless, system designers will need to consider how identification technologies can be incorporated into EP systems as they are developed over the next few years. Consideration will need to be given to where the identification codes are included in a database (and how they are implemented, if a third party dataset is used), as well as how the EP software would drive a barcode/RFID scanner.

At EP innovator sites such as Winchester in the UK, the need to have a physical connection to ward workstations initially limited the usefulness of the EP system. Peripatetic activities, such as <u>electronic medicines administration</u> at the patient's bedside, were simply not feasible in a busy acute setting, regardless of the hardware used. However, the growth of <u>wireless network</u> technology over the past decade has meant that EP software can be accessed from remote wireless units, be they <u>laptop PCs</u>, <u>tablet PCs</u> or trolley-type <u>terminals</u>. Thus, wireless networks have enabled <u>near patient clinical activities</u> such as real-time prescribing during a consultant ward round, and <u>electronic medicines administration</u> by nursing staff. Wireless networks are also the way in which other EP system near-patient services will be facilitated in the future. These will include services such as <u>medicines review</u>, <u>health education</u>, <u>clinical trial</u> management and <u>clinical audit</u>, as discussed in Chap. 6. It is to be hoped that future refinements of wireless network technology – especially in the areas of data transmission and privacy – will be beneficial in developing expanded EP system features in a reliable and scaleable manner.

Issues and Limitations with Quantitative Research on EP Systems

As well as the way in which hardware, software and communications technologies will affect the development of EP systems in future, consideration also needs to be given to the way EP systems are evaluated to assess their effects on organizational efficiency and risk management within a healthcare provider organization.

While a number of large quantitative studies have been carried out in the US, there are very few quantitative data about EP system benefits for UK implementations. While qualitative reports have been published for a number of UK EP implementations [42–44], only one centre – Charing Cross Hospital, London – has undertaken a prospective systematic quantitative analysis of benefits [5]. However, in recent years, work has been conducted to evaluate the earlier UK implementations [45].

In any case, there are many difficulties associated with the quantitative evaluation of EP system benefits. There are issues concerning the design and power of clinical informatics studies, such as those that would be designed to assess EP systems [46], which have been discussed in Chap. 4. In addition, a number of issues have emerged during the actual conduct of EP system evaluation studies. These have included:

(a) the <u>subjectivity of reviewers</u> in the evaluation of adverse events and <u>medication errors</u> in these studies;

(b) the lack of parallel studies between units with EP and those without EP in the same hospital;

(c) error detection bias in error reporting, due to the vigilance of researchers and users when evaluating a new system, and,

(d) the extent to which the benefits reported are specific to the working practices of the sites studied. For these reasons, it has been suggested that there should be a formal methodology for validation of EP software, analogous to the process of licensing a new medicine [47]

As a consequence, there is an urgent need for ongoing quantitative analysis of new EP implementations and enhancements of existing systems. Moreover, there is a need for the quantitative evaluation of EP systems to keep pace with the development of the EP systems themselves, so that, as EP systems become more advanced, new benefits are statistically quantified and emerging risk issues are identified in an accurate and timely manner. This represents a huge future workload for EP implementers and health informatics specialists.

There is a particular need for quantitative benefits studies to be conducted on EP implementations in the UK, where the benefits identified are contextualized into the UK clinical setting. The extent to which benefits are offset by confounding factors associated with research methodology or systems design also needs to be evaluated in more detail.

However, quantitative studies, important though they are, are not the only way of evaluating EP systems. Savage et al. [48] have compared a quantitative and a qualitative analysis of an EP system, and found that, while the two processes provided an similar picture of the drug use process, interviews took less time to conduct than retrospective record review (and were therefore more cost-effective), provided more information on the prescribing process, identified two errors that were not found in record review and provided reasons for delayed or omitted administration of medicines.

Political Issues with EP

It is clear that there are various challenges for EP innovation in the future. These include:

(a) The development of advanced EP functionality and comprehensive decision support and, in particular, the various medical device interfaces that will be needed to support these advanced functions in a "closed loop" process.

(b) The adoption of new hardware technologies and communications modalities to support expanded EP applications

(c) Producing objective quantitative data on the operation of EP systems.

As well as these issues, there is the work required to produce a comprehensive informatics infrastructure (i.e. coding and messaging of EP concepts) to support EP system interoperability across a range of healthcare provider settings (see Chap. 5).

The development of these advanced EP function sets will enable health professionals to develop the new paradigms of working practices described in Chap. 6.

However, EP systems are not developed in a vacuum. EP systems are designed and used by individuals who are clinical professionals and healthcare informatics specialists within particular healthcare provider settings, in association with particular software vendors, and working in a particular national setting. These factors will provide a context in which an EP system operates, and for this reason, the EP system is not just the computer system itself, but the sum of human-computer interactions, and for this reason, EP systems have been rightly referred to as sociotechnical innovations [1]. Furthermore, these factors also provide sociopolitical constraints to system adoption, and new service developments in healthcare mediated by EP systems will only be developed if the political will exists to adopt them.

There are therefore a number of political issues that need to be addressed during the next decade for EP implementation to gather pace.

These are as follows:

- Engagement of clinical professionals

  IT implementations in all sectors have not had a good record of designing software based firmly on recognized business processes or user needs, or of engaging their users with the proposed system prior to its implementation. Indeed, these two steps are interrelated: if the system is not designed so that it is "fit for purpose" for the actual processes that it supports, it will be correspondingly harder to win users over to using the system. Universal engagement with EP innovation by healthcare professions is an issue on both sides of the Atlantic. The English Connecting for Health program conducted clinician engagement workshops in 2006 [49], but these attracted input from clinical professionals who already had an interest in electronic prescribing. There was – and is – more work to be done to engender interest in a broader constituency of healthcare professionals, in particular professionals who are involved with specialized clinical areas and whose input would be required to design advanced EP functionality in those specialties – for example, oncology, HIV infection treatment or mental health. In the US, it has been claimed that EP systems have only been fully adopted at urban centers of excellence, such as the Brigham & Women's Hospital, Boston, Mass., and that EP systems will not be implemented more universally across the US until there are national drug knowledge resources to support the implementation of such systems by healthcare professionals in more remote areas [50].

- Engagement of a broad coalition of software vendors

  At present, it is generally the case that EP system development is the preserve of specialist software developers. These may be IT personnel within healthcare provider organizations, or smaller, niche commercial organizations. In the UK, two organizations with considerable domain expertise in electronic medicines management (JAC Computer Services Ltd and Ascribe) are companies with a track record of developing and installing pharmacy management software. Currently, while many of the major players in healthcare IT development have established markets in systems such as PAS, order communications, laboratory and pathology systems, which are mature markets and therefore low-risk commercial propositions, few of these large companies have made headway in developing comprehensive EP solutions, either as stand-alone applications or as part of a larger suite of software. This is for a number of reasons, concerned with commercial risk compared to established functional areas, and the availability of pharmaceutical domain expertise to these companies [51]. However, for EP systems to become more widely available, the active involvement of large IT vendors will be required. When larger software vendors become seriously committed to the development of EP solutions, designed to reflect actual healthcare processes, then (a) widespread adoption of EP systems will be facilitated, regardless of the existence of regional or national healthcare IT program, and (b) the resources will be available to drive the development of some of the advanced EP functions described elsewhere in this book.

- Fostering the emergence of national and international standards

  While various international standards exist, or are in the process of being developed, for the storage and coding of medical and pharmaceutical concepts, there is no industry standard for EP system design, against which individual systems can be evaluated. This is undoubtedly due to the fact that EP systems are currently the preserve of a few specialist software houses, and are not currently in widespread use. Some work has already been done in this area, from the perspective of required decision support functions, in the US [52]. Furthermore, regional or national healthcare IT program specifications, such as the NHS Connecting for Health Baseline Specification and Hazard Framework have provided some guidance concerning required functionality, but accepted quality standards, endorsed by relevant industry and professional bodies, are still some way in the future. The task of formulating standards is one that will come to the fore when EP systems are more widely available in first-world healthcare economies.

- Monitoring the efficacy of regional or national healthcare IT programs

  In the face of increasing diversity of available systems, together with a perceived need to rationalize the design process, so that the software for an entire health-care economy is designed in a consistent way by a small number of approved vendors, some countries have adopted a national program approach to healthcare software innovation. England had such a program with the NHS Connecting for Health IT program. However, CfH was publicly criticized for its failure to deliver systems to time and to budget, and was decommissioned in 2011. There were a number of important political factors here. Firstly, some claimed that the effectiveness of the national program was fundamentally flawed by competing commercial interests of IT vendors involved and the sheer scale of the project management process. Secondly, it is possible that the requirement to use CfH software actually stifled EP innovation in some English hospitals [53]. Thirdly, it has been argued that large government-sponsored IT projects suffer from a lack of coordination which undoubtedly hinders their delivery schedule; this argument has been made in the UK for both hospital electronic prescribing [54], and the electronic transfer of prescriptions (eTP) in the community [55], and applies equally to other large public sector IT implementations.

It is essential, therefore, that in future the performance of government-sponsored national IT programs in any healthcare economy is carefully monitored, and that such programs are established with realistic goals and expected outcomes.

Conclusion

Currently, EP systems are in operation within just a small proportion of secondary care healthcare providers around the globe. An initial goal for all involved in EP system design, development and implementation must therefore be the more widespread adoption of EP systems. This may be facilitated by advances in hardware and communications technology, and also the development of robust data coding standards; a study of previous implementations suggests that technological changes in the past have led to the development of today's systems. However, current system functionality has only a proportion of the possible functions that could be mediated by a comprehensive EP system. The development of medical device interfaces and telecommunications applications will enable EP systems to play a role in telecare and near-patient healthcare management for the empowered patient. There is a need to link hospital EP systems with new services providing healthcare in the community, such as clinical homecare, and to determine the part that EP systems will play in innovative technologies, such as smart packaging of medicines, which could revolutionize patient care in future. Thus, as well as their potential for reducing risks associated with medicines management in hospitals, and improving the efficiency of healthcare provider business processes, EP systems also have the potential to play a key part in the management of chronic diseases, with profound effects on long-term healthcare expenditure and patient wellbeing.

References

1. Barber N. Electronic prescribing – safer, faster, better? J Health Serv Res Policy. 2010;15 Suppl 1:64–7.
2. Connecting for Health. E-prescribing functional specification for NHS trusts. 2007. p. 125–6. http://connectingforhealth.nhs.uk/systemsandservices/eprescribing. Accessed in January 2012.
3. Hunt DL, Haynes RB, et al. Effects of computer-based clinical decision support systems on physician performance and patient outcomes. J Am Med Assoc. 1998;280:1339–46.
4. Husch M, Sullivan C, et al. Insights from the sharp end of intravenous medication errors: implications for infusion pump technology. Qual Saf Health Care. 2005;14:80–6.
5. Franklin BD, O'Grady K, et al. The impact of a closed-loop electronic prescribing and administration system on prescribing errors, administration errors and staff time: a before and after study. Qual Saf Health Care. 2007;16:279–84.
6. Goundrey-Smith SJ. IT in practice: how "smart" packaging can help with medication adherence. Pharm J. 2010;285:662–3.
7. Fischer S, Stewart TE, et al. Handheld computing in medicine. J Am Med Inform Assoc. 2003;10:139–49.

8. Bates DW, Gawande AA. Improving safety with information technology. N Engl J Med. 2003;348:2526–34.
9. England Department of Health. Equity and excellence: liberating the NHS. 2010. p. 3. http://www.dh.gov.uk/en/Publicationsandstatistics/Publications/PublicationsPolicyAndGuidance/DH_117353. Accessed in January 2012.
10. England Department of Health. An information revolution. 2010. p. 18. http://www.dh.gov.uk/prod_consum_dh/groups/dh_digitalassets/@dh/@en/documents/digitalasset/dh_120598.pdf. Accessed in January 2012.
11. Shane R. Computerised physician order entry: challenges and opportunities. Am J Health Syst Pharm. 2002;59:286–8.
12. Knaup P, Bott O, et al. Electronic patient records: moving from islands and bridges towards electronic health records for continuity of care. Methods Inf Med. 2007;46 Suppl 1:34–46.
13. Ueckert F, Goerz M, et al. Empowerment of patients and communication with healthcare professionals through an electronic health record. Int J Med Inform. 2003;70:99–108.
14. Stewart SF, Switzer JA. Perspectives on telemedicine to improve stroke treatment. Drugs Today (Barc). 2011;47:157–67.
15. McLean S, Chandler D, et al. Telehealthcare for asthma: a cochrane review. Can Med Assoc J. 2011;183:E733–42.
16. McLean S, Nurmatov U, et al. Telehealthcare for chronic obstructive pulmonary disease. Cochrane Database Syst Rev. 2011;7:CD007718.
17. Young LB, Chan PS, et al. Impact of telemedicine intensive care unit coverage on patient outcomes: a systematic review and metaanalysis. Arch Intern Med. 2011;171:498–506.
18. Johnston B. UK telehealth initiatives in palliatve care: a review. Int J Palliat Nurs. 2011;17:301–8.
19. Kidd L, Cayless S, et al. Telehealth in palliative care in the UK: a review of the evidence. J Telemed Telecare. 2010;16:394–402.
20. Magann EF, McKelvey SS, et al. The use of telemedicine in obstetrics: a review of the literature. Obstet Gynecol Surv. 2011;66:170–8.
21. Verberk WJ, Kessels AG, et al. Telecare is a valuable tool for hypertension management, a systematic review and meta-analysis. Blood Press Monit. 2011;16:149–55.
22. Anker SD, Koehler F, et al. Telemedicine and remote management of patients with heart failure. Lancet. 2011;378:731–9.
23. Costa BM, Fitzgerald KJ, et al. Effectiveness of IT-based diabetes management interventions: a review of the literature. BMC Fam Pract. 2009;10:72.
24. Ekeland AG, Bowes A, et al. Effectiveness of telemedicine: a systematic review of reviews. Int J Med Inform. 2010;79:736–71.
25. Gaikwad R, Warren J. The role of home-based information and communications technology interventions in chronic disease management: a systematic literature review. Health Informatics J. 2009;15:122–46.
26. Vitacca M, Mazzu M, et al. Sociotechnical and organisational challenges to wider e-health implementation. Chron Respir Dis. 2009;6:91–7.
27. Woo C, Guihan M, et al. What's happening now! Telehealth management of spinal cord injuries/disorders. J Spinal Cord Med. 2011;34(3):322–31.
28. Koch S, Hagglund M. Health informatics and the delivery of care to older people. Maturitas. 2009;63:195–9.
29. Eron L. Telemedicine: the future of outpatient therapy. Clin Infect Dis. 2010;51 Suppl 2:S224–30.
30. Mc William S. How mobiles and pharmacy are set to revolutionise chronic disease treatment. Pharm J. 2006;276:7–8.
31. Anhoj J, Moldrup C. Feasability of collecting diary data from asthma patient mobile phones and SMS (short message service): review analysis and focus group evaluation from a pilot study. J Med Internet Res. 2004;6:e42.
32. Farmer AJ, Gibson OJ, et al. A randomised controlled trial of the effect of real-time telemedicine support on glycaemic control in young adults with type 1 diabetes. Diabetes Care. 2005;28:2697–702.

33. Gammon D, Arsand E, et al. Parent-child interaction using a mobile and wireless system for blood glucose monitoring. J Med Internet Res. 2005;5:e57.

34. Di Giacomo P, Ricci FL. Generic data modelling and use of XML standard for home telemonitoring of chronically ill patients. Stud Health Technol Inform. 2002;90:163–7.

35. Payne N. The National Clinical Homecare Association. Presented at the National Clinical Homecare Association Conference. Birmingham, UK. 2011. http://www.clinicalhomecare.co.uk/images/stories/documents/presentations/nick_payne.pdf. Accessed in May 2012.

36. Hackett M. Homecare medicines: towards a vision for the future. England Department of Health. 2010. p 6–18. http://cmu.dh.gov.uk/homecare-medicines-review-group. Accessed in January 2012.

37. Hackett M. Homecare medicines: towards a vision for the future. England Department of Health. 2010. p. 10, 51. http://cmu.dh.gov.uk/homecare-medicines-review-group. Accessed in January 2012.

38. Goundrey-Smith SJ. Pharmacy robots in UK hospitals: benefits and implementation issues. Pharm J. 2008;280:599–602.

39. Wind K, Thorp G. E-coding – enhancing supply from manufacturer to patient. Hosp Pharm. 2002;9:240–2.

40. Department of Health Coding for success – simple technology for safer patient care. England Department of Health. London; 2007. p. 17. http://www.dh.gov.uk/en/Publicationsandstatistics/Publications/PublicationsPolicyAndGuidance/DH_066082 . Accessed in May 2012.

41. Adcock H. RFID raises issues associated with privacy and data collision. Hosp Pharm. 2006;13:138.

42. Gray S, Smith J. Practice report – electronic prescribing in Bristol. Healthc Pharm. 2004; August:20–2.

43. Curtis C, Ford NG. Paperless electronic prescribing in a district general hospital. Pharm J. 1997;259:734–5.

44. Foot R, Taylor L. Electronic prescribing and patient records – getting the balance right. Pharm J. 2005;274:210–2.

45. Cornford T, Savage I, Jani Y, et al. Learning lessons from electronic prescribing implementations in secondary care. Stud Health Technol Inform. 2010;160:233–7.

46. Trent Rosenbloom S. Approaches to evaluating electronic prescribing. J Am Med Inform Assoc. 2006;3:399–401.

47. Summers V. Association of Scottish chief pharmacists. Electronic prescribing – the way forward. Pharm J. 2000;265:834.

48. Savage I, Cornford T, Klecun E, Barber N, Clifford S, Franklin BD. Medication errors with electronic prescribing (EP): two views of the same picture. BMC Health Serv Res. 2010;10:135.

49. Hammond B. Electronic prescribing – developing the solution. Hosp Pharm. 2007;14:221–4.

50. Miller RA, Gardner RM, et al. Clinical decision support and electronic prescribing systems: a time for responsible thought and action. J Am Med Inform Assoc. 2005;12:403–9.

51. Goundrey-Smith SJ. Is electronic prescribing a holy grail? Pharm J. 2004;272:412.

52. Teich JM, Osheroff JA, Pifer EA, The CDS Expert Review Panel. Clinical decision support in electronic prescribing: recommendations and an action plan. J Am Med Inform Assoc. 2005;12:365–76.

53. Swanson D. Electronic prescribing – "I wannit and I wannit now!". Hosp Pharm. 2007;14:210.

54. Karr A, Farrell J. Will we ever get a coordinated approach to electronic prescribing? Hosp Pharm. 2003;10:186.

55. Goundrey-Smith SJ. eTP – will we ever get it together? Pharm J. 2007;279:560.

Appendix

Published Worldwide Experience
of Hospital Electronic Prescribing

Location	Literature references
Boston, USA	Bates DW, Leape L, et al. J Am Med Assoc. 1998;280:1311–6 (and other references)
Pennsylvania, USA	Koppel R, Metlay JD, et al. J Am Med Assoc. 2005;293:1197–203
North Carolina, USA	Spencer DC, Leininger A, et al. Am J Health Syst Pharm. 2005;62:416–9
Tennessee, USA	Fitzhenry F, Peterson JF, et al. J Am Med Informat Assoc. 2007;14:756–64
Indiana, USA	Tierney WM, Miller ME, et al. J Am Med Assoc. 1993;269:379–83
Salt Lake City, USA	Evans RS, Pestotnik SL, et al. New Eng J Med. 1998;338:232–8 (and other references)
Ohio, USA	Mekhjian HS, Kumar RR, et al. J Am Med Informat Assoc. 2002;9:529–39
Bristol, England	Gray S, Smith J. Healthcare Pharm. 2004;August:20–22
Burton on Trent, England	Curtis C, Ford NG. Pharm J. 1997;259:734–5
Wirral, England	Farrar K. Pharm J. 1999;263:496–501 (and other references)
Ayr, Scotland	Fowlie F, Bennie M, et al. Pharm J. 2000;265(Suppl):R16
Sunderland, England	Foot R, Taylor L. Pharm J. 2005;274:210–12
Birmingham, England	Nightingale PG, Adu D, et al. Br Med J. 2000;320:750–3
London, England (University College Hospital)	Shulman R, Singer M, et al. Crit Care. 2005;9:R516–21
London, England (Charing Cross Hospital)	Dean Franklin B, O'Grady K, et al. Qual Saf Health Care. 2007;16:279–84 (and other references)
London, England (Institute of Child Health, UCH)	Jani YH, Ghaleb MA, et al. J Pediatr. 2008;152:214–8
Stockholm, Sweden	Sjoborg B, Backstrom T, et al. Int J Med Inform. 2007;76:497–506 (and other references)
Heidelberg, Germany	Seidling HM, Al Barmawi A, et al. Eur J Clin Pharmacol. 2007;63:1185–92
Madrid, Spain	Delgado Silveira E, Soler Vigil M, et al. Farm Hosp. 2007;31:223–30
Valencia, Spain	Llopis Salvia P, et al. Farm Hosp. 2003;27:231–9
South Australia, Australia	Bollen C, Warren J, et al. Aust Fam Physician. 2005;34:283–7 (and other references)

S. Goundrey-Smith, *Principles of Electronic Prescribing*, Health Informatics, DOI 10.1007/978-1-4471-4045-0, © Springer-Verlag London 2012

Index

S. Goundrey-Smith, *Principles of Electronic Prescribing*, Health Informatics,
DOI 10.1007/978-1-4471-4045-0, © Springer-Verlag London 2012

Printed by Printforce, the Netherlands